高等院校药学类专业双语实验教材

分析化学双语实验

主　编　丁瑞芳　段　煜

副主编　魏开芳　高桂花　王晓红　张敏娜

编　者　（以姓氏笔画为序）

丁瑞芳（济宁医学院）	王利涛（济宁医学院）
王晓红（潍坊医学院）	任　强（济宁医学院）
刘潇潇（潍坊医学院）	张敏娜（济宁医学院）
周采菊（济宁医学院）	段　煜（潍坊医学院）
高桂花（济宁医学院）	程忠哲（潍坊医学院）
魏开芳（济宁医学院）	

中国健康传媒集团

中国医药科技出版社

内 容 提 要

　　本教材是"高等院校药学类专业双语实验教材"之一。本套教材编者主要来自济宁医学院和潍坊医学院。为适应医药行业国际化对药学类人才的需求，结合目前大学生英语水平普遍较高的特点，本套教材采用英汉双语编写。本教材共五部分，包括分析化学实验基本知识、基础实验、设计性实验、大型分析仪器仿真操作和附录。

　　本教材供高等医药院校药学类专业教学使用，同时也可供从事药物研究与开发的工作人员参考使用。

图书在版编目（CIP）数据

分析化学双语实验 / 丁瑞芳，段煜主编. —北京：中国医药科技出版社，2019.1
高等院校药学类专业双语实验教材
ISBN 978-7-5214-0728-0

Ⅰ. ①分… Ⅱ. ①丁… ②段… Ⅲ. ①分析化学–化学实验–双语教学–高等学校–教材
Ⅳ. ①O652.1

中国版本图书馆 CIP 数据核字（2019）第 010764 号

美术编辑　陈君杞
版式设计　易维鑫

出版　**中国健康传媒集团** | 中国医药科技出版社
地址　北京市海淀区文慧园北路甲 22 号
邮编　100082
电话　发行：010-62227427　邮购：010-62236938
网址　www.cmstp.com
规格　787×1092mm　$\frac{1}{16}$
印张　10 $\frac{1}{4}$
字数　215 千字
版次　2019 年 1 月第 1 版
印次　2021 年 9 月第 2 次印刷
印刷　北京市密东印刷有限公司
经销　全国各地新华书店
书号　ISBN 978-7-5214-0728-0
定价　**29.00 元**

前　言

分析化学是高等医药教育药学类专业的必修专业基础课,具有实践性较强的特点。分析化学实验在分析化学的教学中占有极其重要的地位,是全面理解并掌握分析化学课程的重要环节,也是培养应用型药学人才不可缺少的一部分。

本教材在编写过程中,编者参照了教育部高等医药院校药学类专业教学指导委员会《药学类专业教学质量国家标准》(2015)和高等医药院校药学类专业《分析化学及分析化学实验大纲》,重点强调分析化学的基本理论知识、科学的思维方法和基本实验技能训练。本教材包括分析化学实验基本知识、基础实验、设计性实验、大型分析仪器仿真操作和附录,共五部分内容。旨在通过严格、系统的实验技能训练,培养学生严谨、实事求是的科学态度以及分析问题、解决问题的能力,为学习药物分析等后修课程和以后从事医药卫生工作奠定良好的基础。

为适应医药行业国际化对药学类人才的需求,本教材采用英汉双语编写。所有编者十多年来一直参与和探索分析化学双语实验教学,通过推行双语实验教学,学生可以掌握分析化学专业核心词汇,培养学生英文文献资料的阅读能力,为将来继续学习奠定基础。

本教材编者主要来自济宁医学院和潍坊医学院,编写分工如下。丁瑞芳(第二部分实验二十至二十一、二十六)、段煜(第三部分,第四部分,附录一)、魏开芳(第二部分实验三至六、附录二至四)、高桂花(第二部分实验七至八、二十二至二十三)、王晓红(第二部分实验九、二十八)、张敏娜(第二部分实验十、十二、十六、二十七)周采菊(第二部分实验十八至十九、二十四)、刘潇潇(第二部分实验十七)、任强(第二部分实验十三至十五、二十五)、王利涛(第一部分、第二部分实验一至二)和程忠哲(第二部分实验十一)。

本教材供高等医药院校药学类专业教学使用,同时也可供从事药物研究与开发的工作人员参考。

本教材是所有编者对多年来双语实验教学的总结。感谢所有编者对本教材的辛勤付出及其所在院校领导的支持。教材中难免存在疏漏与不当之处,敬请读者批评指正。

编　者

2018 年 9 月

目　录

第一部分　分析化学实验基本知识

分析化学实验是一门以实践为基础的课程，是药学及相关专业的实验必修课，主要培养学生严谨的实验作风，实事求是的科学态度，正确地分析问题、解决问题的能力。

一、实验室守则

1. 实验室内应保持安静，严禁大声喧哗、吵闹，遵守秩序。
2. 实验前认真做好预习，了解实验的目的和原理，熟知每个操作步骤，并计划好整个实验应该使用的仪器及其操作程序。
3. 实验过程中，爱护仪器设备，节约药品，严禁粗心大意或浪费药品试剂，如发生事故应及时报告。
4. 实验室台面应随时保持整洁，公用试剂用完后立即放回原处。
5. 仪器使用严格遵守操作规程，发现故障或有损坏立即报告，不得擅自动手检修。
6. 实验室水槽禁止排放具腐蚀性和剧毒液，所有实验用的废弃物应倒入垃圾筒内。
7. 实验室内，水龙头、照明灯和电器应随用随关；易燃品不能直接加热，并要远离火源操作和放置。
8. 实验完毕，实验台面整理干净，并检查仪器、物品以及水、电、煤气。
9. 实验室内一切物品，未经实验室负责教员批准，严禁携带出室外。
10. 值日生负责打扫实验室卫生，最后离开实验室前应认真、负责地进行全面检查，严防事故发生。

二、实验室安全知识

在分析化学实验中，经常使用水、电、易损的玻璃仪器或精密分析仪器以及一些具有腐蚀性甚至易燃、易爆或有毒的化学试剂。为预防分析化学实验中化学药品中毒，操作过程中的烫伤、割伤、腐蚀等危害人身安全的各种因素和燃气、高压气体、高压电源、易燃易爆化学品可能产生的火灾、爆炸及漏水等事故，必须严格遵守实验室的安全规则。

1. 实验室内严禁饮食、吸烟，防止化学试剂入口，实验完毕后必须洗手。
2. 使用 KCN、As_2O_3、$HgCl_2$ 等剧毒品时要特别小心，用过的废物、废液不可乱扔、乱倒，要回收或加以特殊处理。
3. 使用浓酸、浓碱及其他具有强烈腐蚀性的试剂时，操作要小心，防止溅伤和腐蚀皮肤、衣物等。稀释浓酸时（尤其是浓硫酸），应将浓酸沿玻璃棒慢慢倒入水中，切勿反向。

4. 使用易挥发的有毒或有强烈腐蚀性的液体和气体，要在通风橱中操作。如不小心溅到皮肤和眼内，应立即用水冲洗，然后用 5%碳酸氢钠溶液（酸腐蚀时采用）或 5%硼酸溶液（碱腐蚀时采用）冲洗，最后用水冲洗。溅到实验台或地面上要用水稀释后擦掉。

5. 使用高压气体钢瓶时，要严格按操作规程进行操作。例如在原子吸收光谱实验室中所用的各种火焰，其点燃与熄灭的原则是：先开助燃气，再开燃气；先关燃气，再关助燃气（即燃气按"迟到早退"原则开启）。乙炔钢瓶应存放在远离明火、通风良好、温度低于35℃的地方。钢瓶在更换前需保持一部分压力。

6. 在仪器分析实验室中，要在阅读仪器操作规程后或经教师讲解后再动手操作仪器。不要随便拨弄仪器，以免损坏或发生其他事故。

7. 使用自来水后要及时关闭阀门，遇停水时要立即关闭阀门，以防来水后发生跑水，离开实验室之前应再检查自来水阀门是否完全关闭（使用冷凝器时较易忘记关闭冷却水）。

8. 如果发生烫伤或割伤，可先在实验室进行简单处理，然后尽快去医院进行医治。

9. 实验过程中万一起火，不要惊慌，应尽快切断电源或燃气源，用石棉布或湿抹布熄灭（盖住）火焰。密度小于水的非水溶性有机溶剂着火时，不可用水浇，以防止火势蔓延。电器着火时，不可用水冲，以防触电，应使用干冰或干粉灭火器进行灭火。衣服着火时，切忌奔跑，应就地躺下滚动，或用湿衣服在身上抽打灭火。

10. 实验室应保持室内整齐、干净。不能将毛刷、抹布扔在水槽中。保持水槽清洁，禁止将固体废弃物、玻璃碎片等扔入水槽内，以免造成下水管道堵塞。此类物质以及废纸屑等应放入废纸箱或实验室规定放的地方。废酸、废碱等小心倒入废液缸（或塑料提桶内），切勿倒入水槽内，以免腐蚀下水管道。

三、仪器保管及使用的一般规则

1. 实验之前按实验课本上的仪器目录清点清楚，如有缺损及时报告老师，登记补领。

2. 自己保管使用的仪器应有序的摆放，根据每次实验实际需要取出仪器，用完后洗刷干净后放回原处，不能留在实验台上。

3. 每次临时使用的仪器，用完后洗刷干净放在原处，不能放入自己的实验橱内。

4. 精密贵重仪器，应严格按照操作规程使用，未明确用法之前不能随意动仪器。仪器如有故障，及时报告老师。

5. 不准随便使用别组的仪器。

四、实验数据的记录、处理和实验报告

1. 实验数据的记录　学生应有专门的实验记录本，并将之标上页码，不得随便撕去任何一页或乱涂乱画。绝不允许将数据记录在小纸片上或随意记在任何地方。

实验过程中所得的各种测量数据、现象和结果应及时、准确并如实地记录下来。记录实验数据时，要有严谨的科学态度、实事求是，切忌夹杂主观因素，绝不能随意拼凑和伪造数据。若发现数据读错、算错而需要改动时，可将该数据用一横线划去，在旁边写上准确的数据。实验记录不能用铅笔书写，应用钢笔、中性笔、圆珠笔书写。

记录实验数据时，保留几位有效数字应和所用仪器的准确程度相适应。有效数字是在

实验中实际能测量到的数字，记录时估读一位，其余均为准确值，如用分析天平称量时，有效数字应精确至 0.0001 g，滴定管和移液管的读数应精确至 0.01 ml。

实验记录上的每一个数据都是测量结果，所以在重复观测时即使数据完全相同也应记录下来。

2. 分析数据的处理　分析化学实验中，测得一组数据 x_1、x_2、$\cdots$、x_n 后，首先将由于明显的原因所导致的与其他测定数据相差过大的数据删去，其次对其中的可疑数据根据 Q 检验法或 Grubbs 法进行取舍，然后算出算数平均值 $\bar{X}$。同时，还应把分析结果的精密度表示出来。一般用相对平均偏差、标准偏差（S）及相对标准偏差（RSD）表示分析结果的精密度。这些是分析化学实验中最常用的几种处理数据的方法。

3. 实验报告

分析化学的实验报告一般包括下列内容。

实验编号_____实验名称_____实验日期_____

1. 目的要求

2. 方法原理

简要清晰地用文字说明，亦可以用化学反应方程式来说明。

3. 操作步骤

一般可用流线图表示，简明扼要写出。

4. 实验数据及其处理

列出本次实验所测得的数据，可应用文字、表格、图形将数据表示出来，并根据实验要求按一定公式计算出分析结果和分析结果的精密度。

5. 问题及讨论

对实验中观察到的现象及实验结果进行分析和讨论。若实验失败，特别是实验结果出现比较大的误差时，应寻找失败原因，总结经验教训，以提高自己分析问题和解决问题的能力。

五、化学试剂的一般知识

化学试剂的规格是以其中所含杂质的多少来划分的，一般分为四个等级，其规格见表 1-1。

表 1-1　化学试剂规格

等级	名称	英文名称	符号	标签标志
一级品	优级纯（保证试剂）	guaranteed reagent	G.R.	绿色
二级品	分析纯（分析试剂）	analytical reagent	A.R.	红色
三级品	化学纯	chemical reagent	C.P.或 P.	蓝色
四级品	实验试剂	laboratorial reagent	L.R.	棕色等
	生物试剂	biological reagent	B.R.或 C.R.	黄色等

在一般分析化学实验中，通常使用 A.R.级的试剂。

此外，还有基准试剂、色谱纯试剂、光谱纯试剂等。基准试剂的纯度相当于或高于优级纯试剂，它可作为滴定分析法的基准物质，也可用于直接法配制标准溶液。色谱纯试剂是指进行色谱分析时使用的标准试剂，在色谱条件下只出现指定化合物的峰，不出现杂质峰。光谱纯试剂专门用于光谱分析，它以光谱分析时出现的干扰谱线的数目及强度来衡量，其杂质含量用光谱分析法已测不出或其杂质含量低于某一限度。

在选择试剂时不要盲目地追求纯度高，而是应根据分析工作的具体情况进行选择。例如在配制铬酸洗液时，仅需工业用的 $K_2Cr_2O_7$ 及工业硫酸即可，若用 A.R.级的 $K_2Cr_2O_7$，必定造成浪费。当然也不能随意降低试剂的规格而影响分析结果的准确度。

第二部分　基础实验

实验一　滴定分析基本操作

一、实验目的

1. 学习容量仪器的洗涤方法。
2. 掌握滴定管、移液管及容量瓶的操作技术。

二、实验原理

在滴定分析中，规范地使用容量器皿及准确测量溶液的体积，是保证良好分析结果的重要因素。为此，必须学习正确地使用容量仪器，如滴定管、移液管及容量瓶等。

三、仪器和材料

仪器　滴定管，移液管，容量瓶。
材料　蒸馏水，凡士林。

四、实验步骤

1. 滴定管　滴定管是进行滴定操作的器皿，用于测量在滴定中所用标准溶液的体积。滴定管分为两种：一种是酸式滴定管，适用于具有酸性或氧化性的溶液；另一种是碱式滴定管，用于碱性溶液，这两种滴定管不能交换使用。酸性滴定管的下端有一个玻璃活塞，碱式滴定管的下端有一个玻璃球。在滴定分析中经常使用 50 ml 的滴定管，可以读到 0.01 ml，注意保留小数点后两位数字。

（1）检查滴定管　在使用滴定管之前，需要对滴定管进行检查，以确保滴定管正常使用。酸式滴定管的检查，关闭酸式滴定管的活塞，将适量水倒入滴定管，保持 2 分钟。观察是否漏液；如果没有，旋转180°，再保持 2 分钟，再观察是否有漏液。碱式滴定管的检查，将 50 ml 蒸馏水倒入滴定管，保持 2 分钟，观察是否有漏液。如果不漏液，可以使用该滴定管。

（2）酸式滴定管活塞涂油　酸式滴定管活塞涂油的目的是防止漏液，确保活塞转动。最常用的润滑剂是凡士林。润滑活塞的方式如图 1-1 所示，将玻璃活塞从活塞套中取出，用滤纸将活塞及活塞套擦干，在活塞的粗端和活塞套的细端分别涂一薄层凡士林，小心不

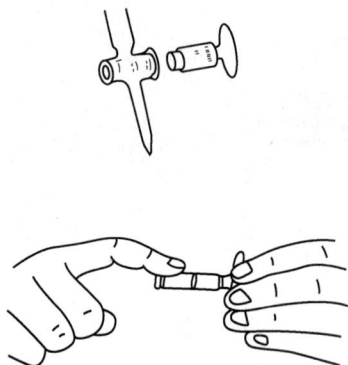

图 1-1 旋塞涂油

要涂在塞孔处以防堵塞孔眼，把活塞插入活塞套内，来回转动数次，直到外面观察时呈透明即可。

（3）洗涤、装液与排气泡　无明显油污的滴定管，直接用自来水冲洗；若有油污可用 5%铬酸洗液 5～10 ml，把滴定管横置，两手平端，转动滴定管直至洗液布满全管。碱式滴定管则应先将橡皮管卸下，把橡皮滴头套在滴定管底部，然后再倒入洗液进行洗涤。污染严重的滴定管，可直接倒入铬酸洗液浸泡几小时。滴定管中附着的洗液用自来水冲洗干净，最后用少量蒸馏水润洗至少 3 次。检测玻璃仪器是否洁净的方法是充满蒸馏水然后放水，只留下一层完整的水膜。如果水聚集成滴则容器仍不干净必须再次清洗。

为了保证装入滴定管溶液的浓度不被稀释，要用该溶液洗滴定管 3 次，每次约用 5～8 ml。清洗时注入溶液后，将滴定管横置，慢慢转动，使溶液流遍全管，然后将溶液自下放出。洗好后可装入溶液，装溶液时要直接从试剂瓶倒入滴定管，不要再经过漏斗等其他容器。

将标准溶液充满滴定管至 0 刻度以上 2～3 cm 米处，并立即打开活塞，使溶液从尖嘴口喷出。检查喷嘴，看是否有气泡。如果有，将滴定管倾斜，迅速打开活塞，让溶液快速流下，反复数次，直至将气泡完全赶出。如为碱式滴定管则可将橡皮管向上弯曲，并在稍高于玻璃珠处，用两手指挤压，使溶液从尖嘴口喷出，气泡即可除尽（见图 1-2）。然后重新装入滴定溶液至 0～0.5 ml 刻度之间，读取凹液面下端的刻度到 0.01 ml，写在记录本上。

（4）滴定　将锥形瓶放置在一张白色纸上或白色的瓷砖上，打开滴定管阀门，滴定液从滴定管中必须慢慢地流出。在滴加滴定液的过程中，必须用一只手不停地摇动锥形瓶，而另一只手控制着旋塞（见图 1-3）。当快到终点时，用洗瓶中少量的蒸馏水清洗瓶壁，继续小心逐滴的滴定，直到出现明显的滴定终点。滴定完毕，等待 2 分钟。记录滴定溶液的体积。

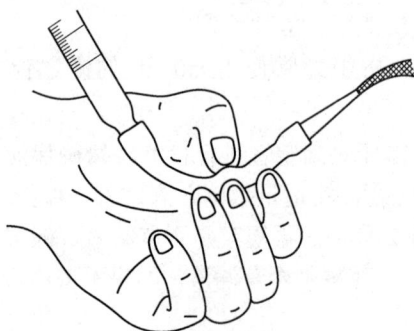

图 1-2　碱式管排除气泡

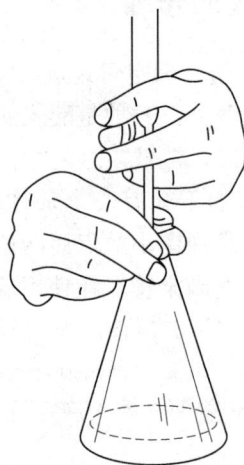

图 1-3　使用酸式滴定管

（5）读数　在滴定完成后，应该记录滴定液的体积，所以首先要读数（包括初读数和终读数），滴定管在读数时要保持竖直，同时眼睛与溶液凹液面在同一水平线，读数精确到 0.01 ml（图 1-4）。滴定读数应记录在原始数据记录本。

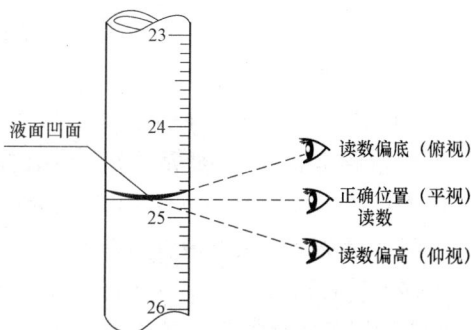

图 1-4　滴定管读数

（6）滴定后的处理　在滴定完成后倒出溶液，并且用蒸馏水洗净，倒置在滴定管架上。在酸式滴定管的活塞和活塞套之间放一张纸。

2. 容量瓶　容量瓶是平底的细长颈梨形容器。颈上有一行小字标识在一个确定温度下的容积，通常温度为 20℃。容量瓶有以下容量：25 ml，50 ml，500 ml，1000 ml。他们用来配制标准溶液到指定容积，同时可以用来借助移液管来得到等分溶液的待分析物质。

（1）容量瓶的检查　在使用容量瓶之前，必须要做以下操作来检查容量瓶是否有渗漏和每个部分是否完好。步骤为：在容量瓶中加入约一半体积的蒸馏水，盖好塞子，倒立，停留大约 2 分钟（图 1-5）。观察有无渗漏，如果没有，转动 180° 停留 2 分钟，再次观察。如果没有渗漏就可以使用。

（2）清洁　一般情况下，如果容量瓶有油污，用 5%铬酸洗液清洗，之后用蒸馏水洗涤。

（3）定容　对固体物质，通常准确称重并放入烧杯，加入约一半容量瓶体积的水来溶解，溶解后将溶液倒入容量瓶（图 1-6），用洗瓶中的蒸馏水洗涤三次烧杯，然后将全部洗涤液转移至容量瓶，在容量瓶 2/3 体积处水平摇匀，接近标线时，要用滴管慢慢滴加蒸馏水，直至溶液的弯月面与标线相切为止，彻底振摇后存放。

对于液体物质，用移液管移取精确体积至容量瓶中，之后按照以上步骤操作。

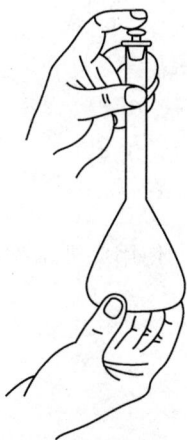

图 1-5　容量瓶的检查

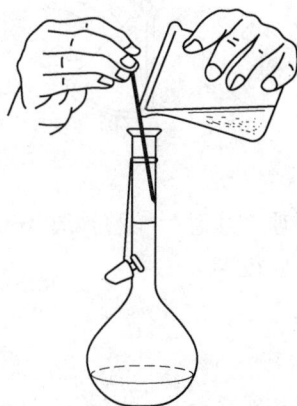

图 1-6　转移溶液

（4）注意事项　注意：①容量瓶不能在干燥箱中干燥或加热来溶解物质；②容量瓶不

能用来长时间存储溶液；③如果容量瓶长时间放置，要在活塞和颈口之间放一片纸。

3. 移液管 移液管有两种：一种是有一个刻度和在特定条件下转移少量恒定体积的溶液（胖肚移液管）；另一种是管上有多个刻度，用来转移不同体积的溶液（刻度或测量移液管）。移液管上有刻度，通常用来转移已指定的不同体积的液体，它在精确工作中不常使用，不作为首选。移液管容积有 1 ml，2 ml，5 ml，10 ml，20 ml，25 ml。

（1）清洗 如果移液管有油污，使用 5%铬酸洗液清洗，之后用蒸馏水洗涤。

（2）转移溶液 在使用移液管时，首先用溶液润洗三次，然后吸至刻度线上 1～2 cm，移液管上端用干燥食指尖封闭（图 1-7），用吸水纸从滴定管下方外部擦拭黏附的液体。通过稍微放松手指的压力直到凹液面刚好达到刻度，此时移液管必须垂直放置，使凹液面与眼睛处于同一水平线。立即按紧食指，移液管的尖端接触容器壁，然后放松食指，液体缓慢流入接收容器。当液体全部流出后，移液管下端与容器侧面壁保持接触 15 s。在排出结束时，移去移液管的尖端，使其不与容器壁接触；保留在移液管中的液体不要通过吹气或其他方式除去。

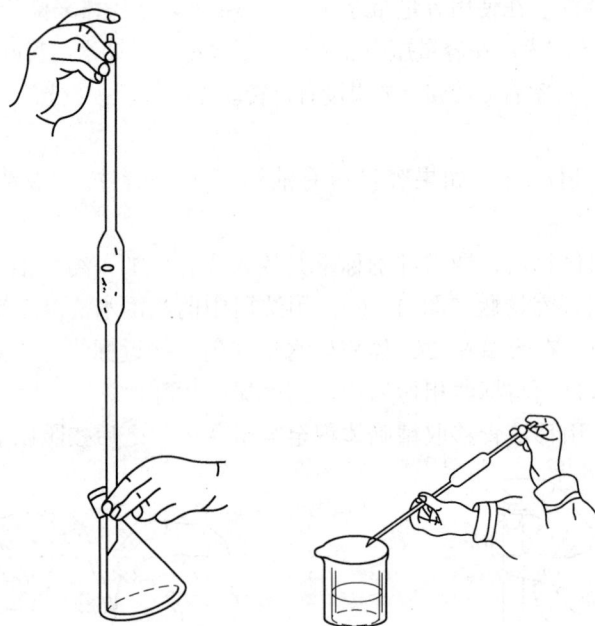

图 1-7 移液管的使用

（3）注意事项 注意：①移液管不能在干燥箱中干燥，使用完要清洗移液管；②当使用以上仪器时，要校准。

Experiment 1　The Basic Operation in Titrimetric Analysis

1. Objective

1.1　Learn the methods of cleaning.

1.2　Master the operation of burette, volumetric flask and pipette.

2. Principle

The most commonly used apparatus in titrimetric analysis are burette, volumetric flask and pipette. Graduated cylinders and weight pipettes are less widely employed. Each of these will be described in turn.

3. Apparatus and Materials

Apparatus: burettes, volumetric flasks, pipettes.

Materials: distilled water, vaseline.

4. Procedures

4.1　Burettes

Burette is a vessel for titration and is used to measure the volume of the standard solution used in titration. Burettes are divided two kinds, one is acid burette, which is used to fill with acidic or oxidation solution, the other is basic burette, which is full of basic solution. Two kinds of burettes can't be exchanged to use. There is a glass stopcock and a jet at the lower end of acidic burette. There is a glass sphere in the bottom of basic burette. The burette of 50 ml is often used in analysis. We can read up to 0.01 ml. So it is possible to read two numbers behind point.

4.1.1　Examination of burette

The following is necessary to check the burette to ensure that the buret is normal before using them. Acid burette inspection: close stopper, and moderate amount of water is pour into the burette, stand for about 2 min. See whether it leak, if not, rotate 180° and stand for another 2 min, see again. Basic burette inspection: pour 50 ml distilled water into the burette, hold for 2 min, and observe whether there is leakage. If it isn't leaky, we can use it.

4.1.2　Lubricants for acid glass stopcocks

The object of lubricating the stopcock of acid burette is to prevent leakage and to ensure smoothness in action. The simplest lubricant is pure Vaseline. To lubricate the stopcock (Fig. 1 − 1), the plug is removed from the barrel and two thin streaks of lubricant are applied to the length of the plug on lines roughly midway between the ends of the bore of the plug, upon

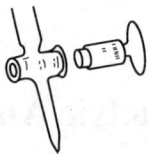

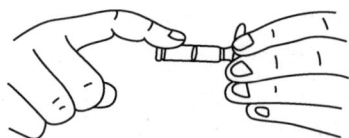

Fig. 1-1 Lubricants for glass stopcocks

replacing in the barrel and turning the tap a few times, a uniform thin film of grease is distributed round the ground joint.

4.1.3 Cleaning, full of solution and remove air bubbles

No obvious oiled burette can be washed directly with tap water. If oiled burette can be washed with 5% chromic acid lotion, place horizontally, the two hands flat, and rotate the buret until the lotion bestrew the tube. The basic burette should remove the rubber tube first, put the rubber tip on the bottom of the burette, and then pour it into the lotion for washing. The severely polluted burette can be poured directly into the chromic acid solution for a few hours. The lotion that is attached to the burette is rinsed off with tap water, and washed at least 3 times with a small amount of distilled water. One test for cleanliness of glass apparatus is that on being filled with distilled water and the water withdrawn, only an unbroken film of water remains. If the water collects in drops, the vessel is dirty and must be cleaned again.

In order to ensure that the concentration of the solution is not diluted, it is necessary to use this solution to wash the burette 3 times, and use 5~8 ml each time. After the solution is injected, the burette place horizontally and slowly turns to allow the solution to flow through the tube, and then the solution is sent out form blow. After washing, the solution can be loaded into the burette, and the solution must be poured directly from the reagent bottle, not through the funnel and other containers.

The standard solution is filled in burette with 2~3 cm above the 0 mark and immediately open the piston to make the solution squirt from the tip of the nozzle. Examine the nozzle to see that no air bubbles enclosed. If there are, tilt the burette, open the piston quickly, and let the solution flow quickly until the jet is completely filled. If it is a basic burette, it can bend the rubber tube up and squeeze it slightly higher than the glass bead, so that the solution can be expelled from the tip of the mouth and the bubbles can be removed (Fig. 1-2). Re-fill, if necessary, to bring the level is between the 0 marks. Read the position of the meniscus to 0.01 ml. Record it in a notebook.

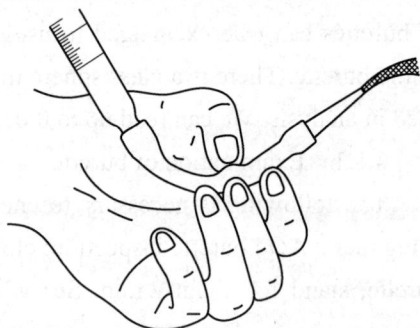

Fig. 1-2 Remove air bubbles for basic burette

4.1.4 Titration

Place the conical flask containing the titrated solution upon a piece of unglazed white paper or a white tile beneath the burette, and run in the titrating solution, the flask must be added slowly from the burette. During the addition of titrating solution, the flask must be constantly rotated with one hand whilst the other hand controls the stopcock (Fig. 1-3). When the end point is coming, wash the walls of the flask down with a little distilled water from a wash bottle, and continue the titration very carefully by adding drop wise titrating solution until the end point of titration is marked. After titration, wait for two minutes; record the volume of titration solution.

4.1.5 Read

After titration, we should record the volume of titration solution, so we first read number (contain of starting and finishing number), burette should place vertical when reading, at this time, solution mark is line with our eyes, read the position of the meniscus to 0.01 ml (Fig. 1 − 4). The burette reading should be taken and recorded in a original data notebook.

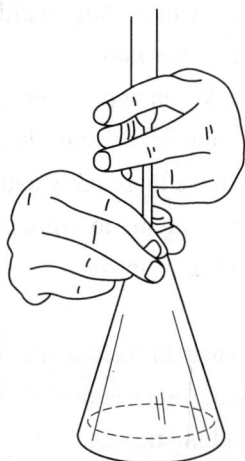

液面凹面

读数偏底（俯视）

正确位置（平视）
读数

读数偏高（仰视）

Fig. 1 − 3   The use of acidic burette   Fig. 1 − 4   Read

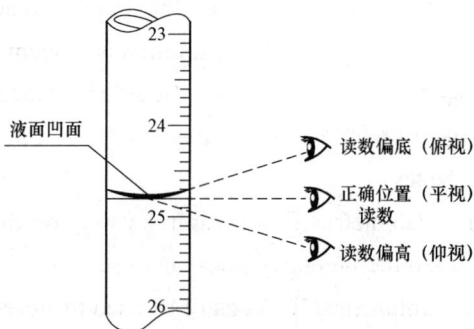

4.1.6 Treatment of titration

Pour off solution after titration, and clean it with distilled water, inverted on the burette holder. Place a piece of paper between plug and barrel of acidic burette.

4.2 Volumetric flasks

A volumetric flask is a flat-bottomed, pear-shaped vessel with a long narrow neck. A thin line etched around the neck indicates the volume that it holds at a certain definite temperature, usually 20 ℃. Graduated flasks are available in the following capacities: 25, 50, 500, 1000 ml. They are employed in making up standard solutions to given volume; they can also be used for obtaining, with the aid of pipettes, aliquot portions of a solution of the substance to be analyzed.

4.2.1 Examination of volumetric flasks

The following is necessary to do before using volumetric flasks, whether volumetric flasks are leaky and each part of volumetric flask is well. The procedure is: half volume distilled water is poured into the volumetric flask, cover the plug and stand upside down, stand for about 2 min (Fig. 1 − 5). See whether it is leak, if not, rotate the stopper for

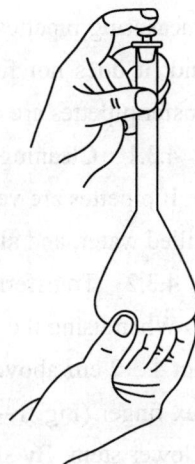

Fig. 1 − 5   The volumetric
flask examination

180° and stand for another 2 min, see again. If it is not leaky, we can use it.

4.2.2　Cleaning

In general, we use 5% chromic acid lotion to clean them if volumetric flasks are very dirty, after that, rinse with distilled water, and allow draining until dry.

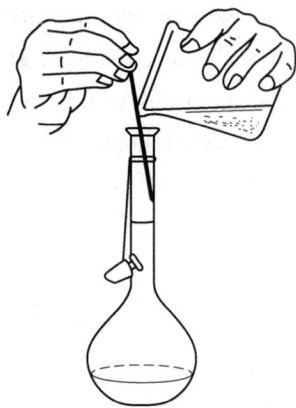

Fig. 1−6　Transfer solution

4.2.3　Fixed volume

For solid substance, we often weigh it correctly, then put it into beaker, adding water about half volume of volumetric flask to dissolve it, after that pour the solution into volumetric flask (Fig. 1−6), wash breaker three times with a little distilled water from a wash bottle, then pour all washings into volumetric flask, and shake well at 2/3 volumetric flask. When approaching the mark line, use the dropper to add distilled water slowly until the meniscus of the solution is tangent to the mark, shake thoroughly and store.

For liquid substance, take an exact volume to volumetric flask with pipette, after that it is to do according to above.

4.2.4　Notes

4.2.4.1　Volumetric flasks can't be dry, or dissolve substance in volumetric flasks by heating.

4.2.4.2　Volumetric flasks can't be used to store solution for a long time.

4.2.4.3　Place a piece of paper between piston and neck of it if volumetric flask may stay for a long time.

4.3　Pipettes

Pipettes are of two kinds: (a) those which have one mark and deliver a small, constant volume of liquid under certain specified conditions (fat belly pipettes); (b) those in which the stems are graduated and are employed to deliver various small volumes at discretion (graduated or measuring pipettes). The pipette has a scale, usually used to transfer the specified volume of liquid: it does not fine wide use in accurate work for which a burette is generally preferred. Transfer pipettes are constructed with capacities of 1ml, 2 ml, 5 ml,, 10 ml, 20 ml and 25 ml.

4.3.1　Cleaning

If pipettes are very dirty, we use 5% chromic acid lotion to clean them. After that, rinse with distilled water, and allow draining until dry.

4.3.2　Transferring solution

When using the pipettes, they are rinsed three times with the liquid, then filled by suction to about 1~2 cm above the mark, and the upper end of pipette is closed with the tip of the dry index finger (Fig. 1−7); any adhering liquid is wiped with absorbent paper from the outside of the lower stem. By slightly relaxing the pressure of the finger until the concave surface reaches the scale, the pipette must be placed vertically so that the concave surface is at the same level as the eye.

Immediately press the index finger, the tip of the pipette touches the wall of the vessel, then relax the index finger, and the liquid slowly flows into the receiving container. When the liquid is all out, the lower end of the pipette stays in contact with the side wall of the container 15 s. At the end of the draining time, the tip of the pipette is removed from contact with the wall of the receptacle; the liquid remaining in the jet of the pipette must not be removed either by blowing or by other means.

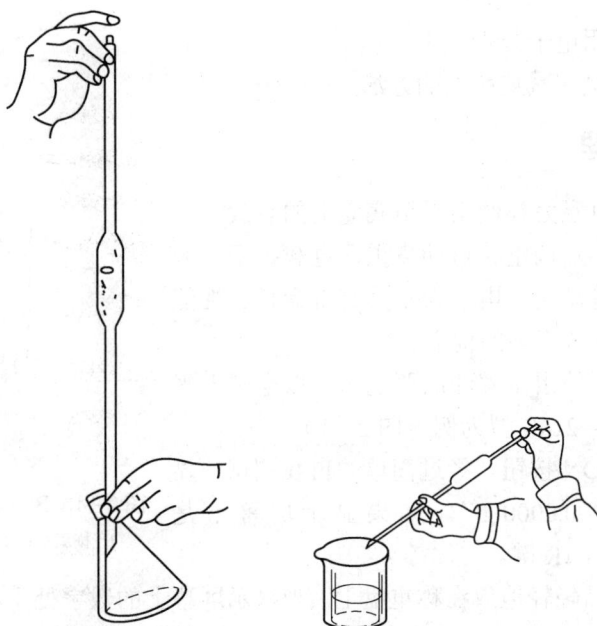

Fig. 1−7   The use of transfer pipettes

4.3.3   Notes

4.3.3.1   Pipettes can't be dried in oven. Cleaning pipettes after using them.

4.3.3.2   The above apparatus must be calibrated when used.

实验二 电子天平与称量练习

一、实验目的

1. 学会正确使用电子分析天平。
2. 熟悉加重称量和减重称量的方法。

二、实验原理

电子天平使用电磁力补偿来平衡底盘上的负载。一般具有自动校准、零点调整、自动皮重、过载指示、故障报警、自动称重等功能。电子天平具有寿命长、性能稳定、操作方便、灵敏度高的优点。

以下是电子天平使用步骤的简要说明，以电子天平的常见赛多利斯 BS-224S 型为例（图 2-1）

1. 开启 点击 ON 按钮，经过简单的自我测试，显示屏幕应该显示 "0.0000 g"。如果显示屏幕不是 "0.0000 g"，按一下 TAR 键。

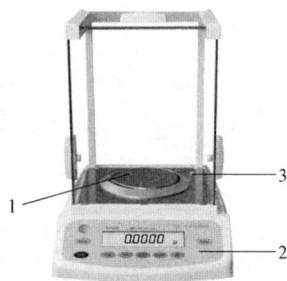

图 2-1 BS-224S 电子天平的示意图
1. 称重盘；2. 控制面板；3. 水平调节

2. 称重 把物品轻轻地放在称重盘上。当显示屏幕上的数字处于稳定状态时，您可以读取并记录称重结果。

3. 扣除皮重 当一个容器放在称重盘上时，它的重量会显示出来。按下 TAR 键，显示出现 0.0000 g，容器的重量已扣除。

4. 关闭 称重完毕，拿走已测量的物品，按 OFF 按钮关闭平衡。

三、仪器和材料

仪器 电子分析天平，称量瓶，烧杯（50 ml 或 100 ml）或锥形瓶（250 ml），不锈钢药品匙。

材料 $K_2Cr_2O_7$

四、实验步骤

1. 直接称重

（1）在称重盘上放置一个清洁的容器。空容器的质量称为皮重。

（2）把化学药品加入到容器中，并读取数字，记下药品质量。

2. 减量称重 适用于易吸水、易氧化或易与二氧化碳反应的物质。

（1）取一定量的粉末样品于称量瓶中，在天平上精密称量，记录称量瓶中样品的重量。

（2）将称量瓶中的样品小心地倒入小烧杯中，再称量一次称量瓶的重量。两者之差即所需样品的重量。

减重称量步骤记录在表 2-1。

3. 称量固定重量（适用于空气中稳定的样品）

（1）在天平上称量出称量纸（或称量瓶、小烧杯等）的重量。

（2）扣除皮重，按 TAR 键，显示出现 0.0000 字样，然后容器的重量被扣除。

（3）用干净的药匙将样品慢慢加入到容器中，直到达到称量要求。

表 2-1　减重法称量

编号	第一次	第二次	第三次
称量瓶 + 样品（g）			
样品（g）			

五、注意事项

1. 为了保护天平不受腐蚀，化学品不应该直接放在称重的平底盘上。
2. 称重范围通常以要求的样品重量为准（1±10%）。
3. 注意样品的重量不应超过天平的最大容量，以避免破坏天平。
4. 除了 ON/OFF 键和 TAR 键，在实验中，学生不允许触摸其余的天平键。

六、思考

1. 在减重法称量中，是否需要设置零点？为什么？
2. 在减重法称量中，可以用药匙添加样品吗？

Experiment 2　Electronic Analytical Balance and Weighing Exercise

1. Objective

1.1　Learn to use analytical balance correctly.

1.2　Grasp weighing method: direct weighing; weighing of fixed weigh; weighing by difference.

2. Principle

An electronic balance uses electromagnetic force compensation to balance the load on the pan. In general, it has automatic calibration, zero adjustment, automatic tare, overload indication, fault alarm, automatic weighing results and other functions. Electronic scale shows good features with a long life, stable performance, easy operation and high sensitivity.

Here is a brief description of the use steps of the electronic balance, take as the common BS-224S type of the electronic balance (see Figure 2 – 1).

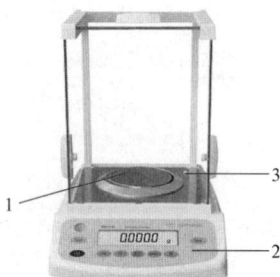

Figure 2 – 1　Schematic diagram of the BS-224S electronic balance

1. weighing pan; 2. control panel; 3. level control

Turn on: Click the ON button, after a brief self-test, the display screen should show "0.0000 g". If the display screen is not 0.0000 g, press the TAR key.

Weighing: Place lightly things on weighing pan. When the digital on the display screen is to be in stable, you may read and record the weighing results.

Deducting the tare: When a container is placed on the pan, its weight can be displayed. Press the TAR key, the display appears 0.0000 g, the weight of the container shall be deducted.

Turn off: When weighing is completed, remove the things to be measured, click OFF button to turn off the balance.

3. Apparatus and Materials

Apparatus: electronic balance, a weighting bottle, a beaker (50 ml or 100 ml) or a conical flask (250 ml), stainless steel medicine spoon.

Materials: $K_2Cr_2O_7$

4. Procedures

4.1　Direct weighing

4.1.1　Place a clean receiving vessel on the balance pan. The mass of the empty vessel is called the tare.

4.1.2　Add the chemical to the vessel and read its mass.

4.2　Weighing by difference

(suitable for absorbing water, oxidation or reaction with carbon dioxide)

4.2.1　First weigh a capped bottle containing dry reagent. Then quickly pour some reagent from the weighing bottle into a receiver.

4.2.2　Cap the weighing bottle and weigh it again. The difference is the mass of reagent delivered from the weighing bottle (Tab.2 – 1).

4.3　Weighing of fixed weight (suitable for the stable sample in air)

4.3.1　Weigh the weighing paper (or weighing bottle, small beaker and so on) alone on the balance.

4.3.2　Deducting the tare: Press the TAR key, the display appears 0.0000 g, and the container weight is deducted.

4.3.3　Add slowly sample with a clean spatula to the container until it meets the weighing requirements.

Table 2 – 1　Weighing by difference

No.	First	Second	Third
Weighting bottle + sample（g）			
Sample（g）			

5. Notes

5.1　To protect the balance from corrosion, chemicals should never be placed directly on the weighing pan.

5.2　Weighing range is generally said to take as the required sample weight of W $(1\pm10\%)$.

5.3　Note the sample's weight should not exceed the maximum capacity of the balance, in order to avoid the damage to balance.

5.4　In addition to the ON/OFF key and TAR key, students are not allowed to touch the rest of the balance keys in this experiment.

6. Questions

1. In weighing by difference, does the zero point need to be set? Why?

2. In the process of weighing by difference, can add sample with medicine spoon?

实验三　0.1 mol/L HCl 标准溶液的配制和标定

一、实验目的

1. 掌握用无水碳酸钠作为基准物质标定盐酸溶液的原理和方法。
2. 正确判断混合指示剂甲基红－溴甲酚绿的滴定终点。
3. 掌握酸式滴定管的操作。

二、实验原理

　　市售盐酸是一种无色透明的氯化氢水溶液，容易挥发，大约含 36%～38% 的 HCl。因此不能直接配制，可采用间接法来配制 0.1 mol/L 盐酸溶液，首先配制一个大约浓度的溶液，然后用基准物质标定。

　　有许多基准物质可以用于 HCl 溶液的标定，如无水碳酸钠、硼砂等。我们用无水碳酸钠作为基准物质，甲基红－溴甲酚绿混合溶液作为指示剂，在滴定终点颜色从绿色变为深紫色。

　　滴定反应可以用下面的公式表示：

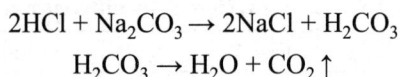

$$2HCl + Na_2CO_3 \rightarrow 2NaCl + H_2CO_3$$
$$H_2CO_3 \rightarrow H_2O + CO_2\uparrow$$

三、仪器和材料

　　仪器　量筒（10 ml），试剂瓶（1000 ml），酸式滴定管（25 ml），锥形瓶（250 ml），电子分析天平。

　　材料　无水 Na_2CO_3 基准物质，浓 HCl（36%～38%），甲基红–溴甲酚绿试剂。

四、实验步骤

　　1. 0.1 mol/L HCl 溶液的配制　用小量筒取 9 ml 浓 HCl 转移至洁净带塞玻璃瓶中，用蒸馏水稀释至 1000 ml 并振摇使之混匀。

　　2. 用无水 Na_2CO_3 标定 0.1 mol/L HCl 溶液　精确称取在 270℃～300℃ 下干燥至恒重的无水 Na_2CO_3 基准物质 0.12 g，用 25 ml 蒸馏水溶解，加入 4～5 滴甲基红–溴甲酚绿溶液，用 0.1 mol/L HCl 滴定至颜色从绿色变为紫红色。煮沸溶液两分钟后冷却至室温，并继续滴定直至溶液由绿色变为深紫色。记下读数。

　　再重复滴定两次。

HCl 溶液浓度可由下列公式计算：

$$C_{\mathrm{HCl}} = \frac{W_{\mathrm{Na_2CO_3}}}{V_{\mathrm{HCl}} \times \dfrac{M_{\mathrm{Na_2CO_3}}}{2000}}$$

$$M_{\mathrm{Na_2CO_3}} = 106.0$$

五、注意事项

1. Na_2CO_3 易吸水，称量速度要快。

2. pH 在终点附近变化不显著，终点变化不敏锐，因为形成了 $Na_2CO_3 - NaHCO_3$ 缓冲溶液，所以我们必须煮沸 2 min 来破坏缓冲溶液，然后冷却至室温，再继续滴定。

六、思考

1. 描述如何配制 1000 ml 0.1 mol/L 盐酸溶液？

2. 锥形瓶是否需要干燥？实验中蒸馏水的用量是否需要精确？

3. 当滴定接近完成时为什么溶液要煮沸？为什么溶液要冷却到室温？

4. 在这个实验中如果需要消耗 23 ml 0.1 mol/L 盐酸标准溶液，要称量多少无水 Na_2CO_3？

Experiment 3　Preparation and Standardization of Standard 0.1 mol/L Hydrochloric Acid Solution

1. Objective

1.1　Master the principle and method of using anhydrous sodium carbonate as primary standard substance to standardize hydrochloric acid solution.

1.2　Judge correctly end point of the mixed indicator of methyl red-bromocresol green solution.

1.3　Master the operation of the acid burette.

2. Principle

The commercial hydrochloric acid is a colorless and transparent aqueous solution of hydrogen chloride. It is easy to volatize and contains about 36% to 38% (*w/w*) of HCl. So the standard solution can not be prepared directly, so indirect method is adopted for the preparation of 0.1 mol/L hydrochloric acid. That is, an solution of the approximate concentration is firstly prepared, and then standardized with primary standard substance.

There are a number of primary standards used as standardization for hydrochloric acid, such as anhydrous sodium carbonate, borax, and so on. We use anhydrous sodium carbonate as primary standard and methyl red-bromocresol green mixed solution as indicator. The color changes from green to dark purple at the end point.

The reaction of titration may be represented in the following equation:

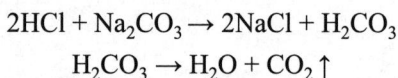

$$2HCl + Na_2CO_3 \rightarrow 2NaCl + H_2CO_3$$
$$H_2CO_3 \rightarrow H_2O + CO_2 \uparrow$$

3. Apparatus and Materials

Apparatus: cylinder (10 ml), glass reagent bottle (1000 ml), acid burette (25 ml), conical flask (250 ml), electronic analytical balance.

Materials: primary standard (anhydrous Na_2CO_3), concentrated hydrochloric acid (36%~38%), methyl red-bromocresol green indicator.

4. Procedures

4.1　Preparation of 0.1 mol/L hydrochloric acid solution

Measure out 9 ml of concentrated hydrochloric acid by a small cylinder, and transfer to a clean glass reagent bottle. Dilute it to 1000 ml with distilled water and thoroughly mix by shaking.

4.2　Standardization of 0.1 mol/L hydrochloric acid with anhydrous sodium carbonate

Weigh out accurately about 0.12 g of primary standard anhydrous sodium carbonate (which has been previously dried at a temperature of about 270 ℃ to 300 ℃ until the weight is constant). Dissolve it with 25 ml of distilled water, and add $4\sim5$ drops of methyl red-bromocresol green solution. Titrate it with 0.1 mol/L hydrochloric acid until the color changes from green to purple-red. Boil the solution for about two minutes, then cool it to room temperature and continue the titration until the color of solution changes from green to dark purple. Set down the reading.

Repeat the standardization for another 2 times.

The concentration of hydrochloric acid can be calculated from the formula:

$$C_{HCl} = \frac{W_{Na_2CO_3}}{V_{HCl} \times \dfrac{M_{Na_2CO_3}}{2000}}$$

$$M_{Na_2CO_3} = 106.0$$

5. Notes

5.1　Na_2CO_3 is easy to absorb water and the weighing process is required rapid.

5.2　pH of solution does not change greatly when the titration is close to the end point due to the forming of $H_2CO_3 - NaHCO_3$ buffer solution. So we have to boil the solution for 2 minutes to break the buffer solution, and then cool it to room temperature and continue the titration.

6. Questions

6.1　How to prepare 1000 ml 0.1 mol/L hydrochloric acid solution.

6.2　Whether the conical flask must be dried and the quantity of distilled water must be accurate during the experiment.

6.3　Why is the solution boiled when titration is nearing completion? Why is the the solution cooled to room temperature?

6.4　If 23 ml 0.1 mol/L hydrochloric acid is required for standardization of hydrochloric acid in this experiment, how many grams of anhydrous sodium carbonate must be weighed out?

实验四　混合碱的含量测定

一、实验目的

1. 掌握混合碱的测定方法。
2. 了解双指示剂法的原理和应用。

二、实验原理

混合碱系指 Na_2CO_3 与 NaOH 或 Na_2CO_3 与 $NaHCO_3$ 的混合物,可用强酸采用"双指示剂法"进行测定。根据滴定过程中 pH 值的变化,选用两种指示剂,即酚酞和甲基橙来指示终点,这就是通常所说的双指示剂法。

若混合碱是 Na_2CO_3 与 NaOH 的混合物,先以酚酞作指示剂,用 HC1 标准溶液滴定至溶液刚好褪色(或略带粉红色),这是第一化学计量点。此时 NaOH 完全被中和,而 Na_2CO_3 被中和至 $NaHCO_3$ (只中和了一半),其反应为:

$$HCl + NaOH = NaCl + H_2O \qquad 酚酞(红色 \rightarrow 无色)$$
$$HCl + Na_2CO_3 = NaHCO_3 + NaCl \qquad 酚酞(红色 \rightarrow 无色)$$

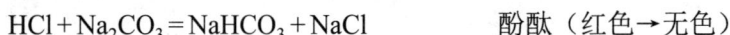

设用去标准酸溶液 V_1 毫升。

再以甲基橙作指示剂,继续用 HCl 标准溶液滴定至溶液呈现橙色,这是第二化学计量点。反应为:

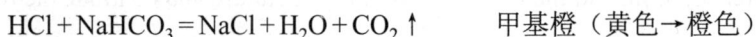

$$HCl + NaHCO_3 = NaCl + H_2O + CO_2 \uparrow \qquad 甲基橙(黄色 \rightarrow 橙色)$$

设此时用去标准酸溶液 V_2 毫升。

样品中各组分的含量可由以下假设来确定。

(1)若 $V_1 > V_2$,样品的组成为 Na_2CO_3 与 NaOH。Na_2CO_3 消耗标准酸的体积为 $2V_2$,NaOH 消耗标准酸的体积为 $(V_1 - V_2)$。根据标准酸的浓度和所消耗的体积,便可算出混合碱中 Na_2CO_3 和 NaOH 的百分数。

(2)若 $V_1 < V_2$,样品的组成为 Na_2CO_3 与 $NaHCO_3$。Na_2CO_3 消耗标准酸的体积为 $2V_1$,$NaHCO_3$ 消耗标准酸的体积为 $(V_2 - V_1)$。根据标准酸的浓度和所消耗的体积,便可算出混合碱中 Na_2CO_3 和 $NaHCO_3$ 的百分数。

三、仪器和材料

仪器　锥形瓶(250 ml),酸式滴定管(25 ml),移液管(20 ml)。
材料　混合碱,盐酸标准溶液(0.1 mol/L),甲基橙指示剂(0.2%),酚酞指示剂(0.2%)。

四、实验步骤

用移液管准确移取 20 ml 混合碱溶液于 250 ml 锥形瓶中,加酚酞指示剂 2～3 滴,以

0.1 mol/L HCl 标准溶液滴定至溶液红色刚好褪去为止，记下 HCl 溶液体积（V_1）。然后再加入 1～2 滴甲基橙指示剂，继续滴定至溶液由黄色恰好变为橙色，记下此时用去 HCl 标准溶液体积（V_2）。重复滴定 2 次。

根据消耗的 HCl 标准溶液的体积，来判断试样的组成，并计算各组分的百分含量。

五、注意事项

以酚酞作为指示剂时，滴定终点溶液红色恰好褪去，这个变化不易判断，需仔细观察。

六、思考

1. 这个实验中还可以用其他指示剂吗？
2. 试推导各组分的计算公式。

Experiment 4　Determination of Mixed Base

1. Objective

1.1　Master the method of the determination of mixed base.

1.2　Learn the principle and application of the double indicator method.

2. Principle

Mixed base refers to the mixture of Na_2CO_3 and NaOH or Na_2CO_3 and $NaHCO_3$, which can be determined with strong acid by "double indicator method". According to the change of pH during the procedure, two indicator, phenolphthalein and methyl orange are usually used to detect the end point. This is generally referred to the double indicator method.

If the mixed base is a mixture of Na_2CO_3 and NaOH, we can use phenolphthalein as indicator in the first step. Titrate the solution by HCl standard solution until the color just fade (or slightly pink), and this is the first stoichiometric point. At this point, NaOH is completely neutralized, while Na_2CO_3 is neutralized to $NaHCO_3$ (half neutralized), the reaction is:

$$HCl + NaOH = NaCl + H_2O \qquad \text{phenolphthalein (red} \rightarrow \text{colorless)}$$
$$HCl + Na_2CO_3 = NaHCO_3 + NaCl \qquad \text{phenolphthalein (red} \rightarrow \text{colorless)}$$

The volume of standard acid solution consumed is V_1 ml.

Then the titration is continued using methyl orange as indicator until the solution exhibits orange, which is the second stoichiometric point. The reaction equation is as following:

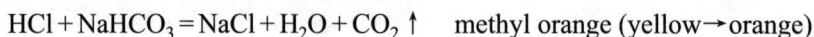

$$HCl + NaHCO_3 = NaCl + H_2O + CO_2 \uparrow \qquad \text{methyl orange (yellow} \rightarrow \text{orange)}$$

The volume of HCl consumed at this point is V_2 ml.

The composition of the sample is determined by the following assumptions.

a. If $V_1 > V_2$, the composition of the sample is Na_2CO_3 and NaOH.

Standard acid volume consumption of Na_2CO_3 is $2V_2$ ml and NaOH is $(V_1 - V_2)$ ml. According to the concentration of acid and the volume, the percentage of Na_2CO_3 and NaOH can be calculated in mixed base.

b. If $V_1 < V_2$, the composition of the sample is Na_2CO_3 and $NaHCO_3$.

The standard acid volume consumption of Na_2CO_3 is $2V_1$ ml and $NaHCO_3$ is $(V_2 - V_1)$ ml. According to the concentration of acid and the volume, the percentage of Na_2CO_3 and $NaHCO_3$ can be calculated in mixed base.

3. Apparatus and Materials

Apparatus: conical flask (250 ml), acid burette (25 ml), pipette (20 ml).

Materials: mixed base, hydrochloric acid standard solution (0.1 mol/L), methyl orange indicator (0.2%), phenolphthalein indictor (0.2%).

4. Procedures

Transfer 20.00 ml mixed alkali solution to a 250 ml conical flask with a pipette, add 2~3 drops of phenolphthalein indicator, and then titrate the solution with 0.1 mol/L HCl standard solution until the red color just faded. Write down the volume (V_1). Then add 1~2 drops of methyl orange indicator, and continue the titration until the color changes from yellow to orange. Write down the HCl standard solution volume (V_2) of this step.

Repeat twice as described above.

According to V_1 and V_2, we can determine the sample composition, and calculate the percentage content of each component.

5. Notes

When we use phenolphthalein as indicator, the red color fades at the end point. This change is not easy to judge, so we must observe carefully.

6. Questions

6.1　What other indicators can be used in this experiment?

6.2　Try to deduce the calculation formula of each component content.

实验五　0.1 mol/L 氢氧化钠标准溶液的配制与标定

一、实验目的

1. 掌握氢氧化钠溶液配制方法及用基准物质邻苯二甲酸氢钾标定标准溶液的方法。
2. 掌握碱式滴定管的操作方法。
3. 学会正确判断酚酞的滴定终点。

二、实验原理

NaOH 会迅速地从空气中吸 H_2O 和 CO_2，一定量的 Na_2CO_3 总是存在：

$$2NaOH + CO_2 \longrightarrow Na_2CO_3 + H_2O$$

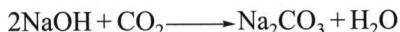

所以配制 0.1 mol/L NaOH 溶液需采用间接配制法。即通常先配制近似浓度的 NaOH 溶液，通过用基准物质标定来获得准确浓度。

有很多方法可以用来配制无碳酸盐的标准 NaOH 溶液，最常用的方法是用饱和 NaOH 溶液来配制。碳酸钠在饱和 NaOH 溶液中不溶解而沉淀下来，吸取上清液并用无 CO_2 的水稀释成近似所需浓度的溶液，再用基准物质标定。

有许多基准酸可用来标定碱性溶液，如含 2 个结晶水的草酸（$H_2C_2O_4 \cdot 2H_2O$）、苯钾酸（C_6H_5COOH）、氨基磺酸（NH_2SO_3H）和邻苯二甲酸氢钾（$KHC_8H_4O_4$）等，目前，邻苯二甲酸氢钾最常用，其反应如下：

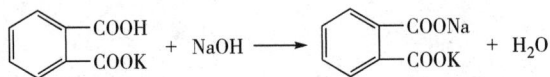

使用酚酞溶液作为指示剂，在滴定终点由于弱酸盐的水解，溶液会略显碱性。

三、仪器和材料

仪器　碱式滴定管（25 ml），锥形瓶（250 ml），量筒（100 ml），烧杯（500 ml），塑料试剂瓶（500 ml），电子分析天平。

材料　氢氧化钠（分析纯），酚酞指示剂。

四、实验步骤

1. 饱和氢氧化钠溶液的配制　在 100 ml 蒸馏水中溶解 120 g NaOH，充分摇匀，冷却溶液并转移到塑料瓶内，溶液在塑料瓶内放置几天使得所有不能溶解在浓 NaOH 溶液中的 Na_2CO_3 沉淀至底部。

2. 0.1 mol/L NaOH 溶液的配制　吸取 2.8 ml 的饱和 NaOH 溶液至一个塑料试剂瓶，加入新沸并放冷的蒸馏水至 500 ml，充分振摇。

3. 0.1 mol/L NaOH 溶液的标定　取约 0.45 g 基准物质邻苯二甲酸氢钾（在 105～110 ℃干燥至恒重），精密称定，每个锥形瓶中加入 30 ml 新沸过并放冷的蒸馏水，轻轻振摇至样品全部溶解，加入 2 滴酚酞指示剂，用 0.1 mol/L NaOH 滴定溶液至粉色，并保持 30 s 不褪色。记录最终读数。再重复 2 次。

根据称量的邻苯二甲酸氢钾的质量和消耗 NaOH 的量计算 NaOH 标准溶液的浓度。

$$C_{NaOH} = \frac{W_{KHC_8H_4O_4} \times 1000}{V_{NaOH} \times M_{KHC_8H_4O_4}}$$

$$M_{KHC_8H_4O_4} = 204.2$$

五、注意事项

1. 氢氧化钠必须在烧杯中称量，不能在称量纸上称量。
2. 每次滴定前，滴定管的液面要调到零。

六、思考

1. 如果中和 23 ml 0.1 mol/L NaOH 溶液，需要多少克邻苯二甲酸氢钾？
2. 如果基准物质邻苯二甲酸氢钾没有预先在 105～110 ℃中干燥，则 NaOH 标准溶液的浓度会有何影响？

Experiment 5 Preparation and Standardization of Standard Solution of 0.1 mol/L Sodium Hydroxide Solution

1. Objective

1.1 Master how to prepare and standardize sodium hydroxide standard solution with potassium acid phthalate primary standard substances.

1.2 Master the operation of the basic burette.

1.3 Learn to judge the end point of phenolphthalein correctly.

2. Principle

Sodium hydroxide can rapidly absorb water and carbon dioxide from the air. A certain amount of sodium carbonate is always present.

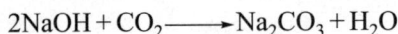

$$2NaOH + CO_2 \longrightarrow Na_2CO_3 + H_2O$$

So indirect method is adopted for the preparation of 0.1 mol/L sodium hydroxide solution. It is customary to prepare sodium hydroxide solution of approximate concentration and then standardize it against a primary standard to obtain the exact concentration.

There are several methods can be used to prepare carbonate-free standard sodium hydroxide solution, and the saturated sodium hydroxide solution method is thought to the most common method. Sodium carbonate is insoluble in the saturated sodium hydroxide solution, and can be precipitated to the bottom of the bottle. Siphon off the clear supernatant liquid and dilute it with carbon dioxide - free water to the approximate concentration, then standardize the standard solution against a primary standard.

There are several primary standard acids to standardize the basic solution, for example, oxalic acid dihydrate ($H_2C_2O_4 \cdot 2H_2O$), benzoic acid (C_6H_5COOH), sulfamic acid (NH_2SO_3H) and potassium acid phthalate ($KHC_8H_4O_4$) etc. At present the last one is preferable, and the reaction is as follows:

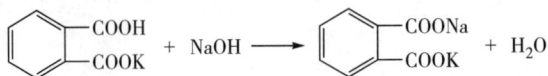

Phenolphthalein solution is used as indicator, the solution at the equivalence point would be slightly alkaline, due to the hydrolysis of the weak acid salt.

3. Apparatus and Materials

Apparatus: basic burette (25 ml) , conical flask (250 ml), cylinder (100 ml), beaker (500 ml), plastic reagent bottle (500 ml), electronic analytical balance.

Materials: NaOH (A.R), phenolphthalein indicator.

4. Procedures

4.1　Preparation of saturated NaOH solution

Dissolve 120 g of NaOH in 100 ml of distilled water, shake well, cool the solution and transfer to a plastic reagent bottle. Allow the solution to stand for several days so that any Na_2CO_3 (which is insoluble in concentrated NaOH) will settle to the bottom.

4.2　Preparation of 0.1 mol/L NaOH solution

Siphon off 2.8 ml of the saturated NaOH solution to a plastic reagent bottle. Add distilled water which is freshly boiled and cooled to make 500 ml, and shake well.

4.3　Standardization of 0.1 mol/L NaOH solution

Weigh out accurately about 0.45 g primary standard potassium acid phthalate (dried at $105\sim110$ ℃ until the weight is constant) to a conical flask, adding 30 ml of distilled water which is freshly boiled and cooled to the flask and shake gently until the sample is dissolved. Add 2 drops of phenolphthalein indicator solution, titrate the solution with 0.1 mol/L NaOH solution to the first permanent pink color, which should persist not less than thirty seconds. Record the final reading. Repeat the standardization twice.

Calculate the concentration of the NaOH standard solution based on the weight of the salt and the final reading of the NaOH.

$$C_{NaOH} = \frac{W_{KHC_8H_4O_4} \times 1000}{V_{NaOH} \times M_{KHC_8H_4O_4}}$$

$$M_{KHC_8H_4O_4} = 204.2$$

5. Notes

5.1　We must weigh sodium hydroxide in a beaker instead of on a piece of paper.

5.2　Adjust liquid level of the burette to zero point before each titration.

6. Questions

6.1　How many grams of potassium acid phthalate is needed if 23 ml of 0.1 mol/L NaOH is required to neutralize it .

6.2　If the primary standard potassium acid phthalate has not been previously dried at a temperature of about 105 ℃ to 110 ℃, the concentration of the NaOH standard solution will be higher or lower?

实验六 阿司匹林的含量测定

一、实验目的

1. 掌握用酸碱滴定法测定阿司匹林的原理及操作。
2. 掌握酚酞指示剂滴定终点的判断。
3. 掌握中性乙醇的配制方法。

二、实验原理

阿司匹林属于芳香族羧基酯类药物，它在水中的溶解度很小，可以在乙醇中用氢氧化钠滴定。反应方程式为：

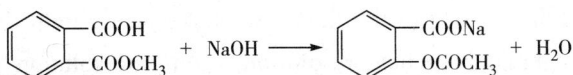

滴定时，溶液的温度要控制在 10 ℃以下，以防止阿司匹林的水解。在滴定终点，反应产物是强碱弱酸盐，由于盐的水解作用，溶液略显碱性。所以在这个滴定中应该使用碱性区变色的指示剂，本实验使用酚酞做指示剂。

三、仪器和材料

仪器 碱式滴定管（25 ml），锥形瓶（250 ml），烧杯（100 ml），量筒（100 ml，10 ml），电子分析天平。

材料 阿司匹林，NaOH 标准溶液（0.1 mol/L），酚酞指示剂，无水乙醇。

四、实验步骤

精确称量三份 0.4 g 阿司匹林置三个洁净并标号的 250 ml 锥形瓶中，加入 10 ml 中性乙醇（对酚酞显中性），然后加入 2～3 滴酚酞指示剂，并用 0.1 mol/L 的 NaOH 标准溶液滴定至出现粉红色，并保持 30 s 不褪色。滴定过程中温度必须低于 10 ℃。

计算公式为：

$$C_9H_8O_4\% = \frac{C_{NaOH} \times V_{NaOH} \times M_{C_9H_8O_4}}{W_{C_9H_8O_4} \times 1000} \times 100\%$$

$$M_{C_9H_8O_4} = 180.2$$

五、注意事项

1. 中性乙醇的配制：在一定量的乙醇中加入 2～3 滴酚酞指示剂溶液，用 0.1 mol/L 的 NaOH 标准溶液滴定直至出现粉红色。

2. 阿司匹林在水中微溶，在乙醇中易溶解，所以乙醇可以作为溶剂，水解反应也可避免。

六、思考

1. 在配制标准酸溶液或标准碱溶液时，如果某溶液已被充分振摇，那后来再使用时，是否需要再次振摇？

2. 根据步骤要求，每份样品称量需要 0.4 g，如果一份样品倒入过多，重量达 0.4537 g，是否需要重新称量？

Experiment 6　Determination of Aspirin

1. Objective

1.1　Master the principle and operation of determination of aspirin with the acid - basic titration.

1.2　Master the end point of the phenolphthalein indicator.

1.3　Master the preparation of neutral alcohol.

2. Principle

Aspirin belongs to the medicines of aromatic carboxylic ester. It has low solubility in water, and can be determined against sodium hydroxide solution in alcoholic media instead of in water. The reaction of titration is:

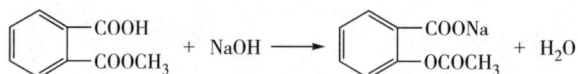

When the titration is carried out, the temperature ought to be controlled below 10 ℃ to avoid hydrolysis reaction. At the equivalence point, the reaction product is the salt of the weak acid and the strong base. The solution would be slightly alkaline due to hydrolysis of the salt. So an indicator of alkaline range ought to be adopted in the titration. Thus phenolphthalein should be used as indicator in the titration.

3. Apparatus and Materials

Apparatus: basic burette (25 ml), conical flask (250 ml), beaker (100 ml), cylinder (10 ml, 100 ml), electronic analytical balance.

Materials: aspirin, standard NaOH solution (0.1 mol/L), phenolphthalein indicator, alcohol anhydrous.

4. Procedures

Weigh accurately about three portions of 0.4 g aspirin into three clean, numbered 250 ml conical flask, add 10 ml of neutral ethanol (for neutralization against phenolphthalein) and 2～3 drops of phenolphthalein indicator solution and titrate with 0.1 mol/L of sodium hydroxide standard solution to the first permanent pink color, which should persist not less than thirty seconds. The temperature must be below 10 ℃ during the titration.

Calculation equation is as following：

$$C_9H_8O_4\% = \frac{C_{NaOH} \times V_{NaOH} \times M_{C_9H_8O_4}}{W_{C_9H_8O_4} \times 1000} \times 100\%$$

$$M_{C_9H_8O_4} = 180.2$$

5. Notes

5.1　Preparation of Neutral Alcohol

Add 2～3 drops of phenolphthalein indicator solution to a required amount of alcohol.Then titrate with 0.1 mol/L sodium hydroxide standard solution until a pink color is obtained.

5.2　Aspirin slightly dissolves in water and freely dissolves in alcohol, so alcohol is selected as solvent and hydrolysis could be avoided.

6. Questions

6.1　If a solution has been shaken fully in preparation of standard acid solution or standard alkali solution, is it necessary to shake again when it is used afterwards？

6.2　According to the procedure, each portion of sample should be weighed about 0.4 g. Now a portion of sample is poured out excessively, its weight is 0.4537 g. Is it necessary to weigh it again?

实验七　0.05 mol/L EDTA 标准溶液的配制与标定

一、实验目的

1. 掌握间接法配制 EDTA 标准溶液的方法。
2. 掌握 EDTA 标准溶液的标定方法。
3. 了解铬黑 T 指示剂终点的判断方法。

二、实验原理

由于 EDTA 在水中的溶解度小，所以通常采用 EDTA 二钠盐配制标准溶液，也称为 EDTA 溶液。EDTA 二钠盐是一种白色结晶性粉末，分子量为 372.26。室温下，100 ml 水中可溶解 11.1 g EDTA 二钠盐。EDTA 标准溶液采用间接法配制，即取适量 EDTA 二钠盐溶于适量水中，摇匀，储存于硬质玻璃瓶中。用 ZnO 或 Zn 为基准物质对其准确浓度进行标定，以铬黑 T 或二甲酚橙作指示剂。

三、仪器和材料

仪器　滴定管（25 ml），锥形瓶（250 ml），容量瓶（500 ml），烧杯（50 ml）。

材料　EDTA 二钠盐，ZnO 基准物质，稀盐酸溶液，甲基红指示剂，氨试液，$NH_3 \cdot H_2O - NH_4Cl$ 缓冲液，铬黑 T 指示剂。

四、实验步骤

1. 0.05 mol/L EDTA 标准溶液的配制　称取 9.5 g EDTA 二钠盐，用适量水溶解后，转移到 500 ml 容量瓶，继续用水稀释至刻度后，摇匀。将配制好的溶液转移至硬质玻璃瓶中储存，待用。

2. 0.05 mol/L EDTA 标准溶液的标定　精密称取在 800 ℃干燥至恒重的 ZnO 约 0.12 g，加稀盐酸 3 ml 使溶解，再加入 25 ml 蒸馏水及 1 滴甲基红指示剂，滴加氨试液至溶液呈现微黄色，再加入 25 ml 蒸馏水、10 ml $NH_3 \cdot H_2O - NH_4Cl$ 缓冲液及 2 滴铬黑 T 指示剂，用 EDTA 溶液滴定至溶液由紫红色变成纯蓝色即为终点。

计算公式：

$$C_{\mathrm{EDTA}} = \frac{W_{\mathrm{ZnO}} \times 1000}{M_{\mathrm{ZnO}} V_{\mathrm{EDTA}}}$$

$$M_{\mathrm{ZnO}} = 81.38$$

五、注意事项

1. EDTA 二钠盐在水中溶解缓慢，需要不断搅拌或者加热来加速溶解。

2. 配制好的 EDTA 溶液应储存于硬质玻璃瓶中，否则，EDTA 会与瓶体中的金属离子反应，进而影响 EDTA 的浓度。

3. 滴定过程不能过快，尤其需注意接近滴定终点时应逐滴加入滴定剂，并不断振摇。

六、思考

1. 加入 $NH_3 \cdot H_2O - NH_4Cl$ 缓冲液的作用是什么？

2. 实验步骤中为什么需要加入甲基红指示剂后滴加氨试液至溶液呈现微黄色？

Experiment 7 Preparation and Standardization of 0.05 mol/L EDTA Standard Solution

1. Objective

1.1 Master the preparation of EDTA standard solution by indirect method.

1.2 Master the standardization method of EDTA standard solution.

1.3 Understand the judgement of the end point by Eriochrome Black T (EBT) indicator.

2. Principle

Due to the low solubility of EDTA in water, $Na_2H_2Y \cdot 2H_2O$ is usually used to prepare standard solution, which is also known as EDTA solution. $Na_2H_2Y \cdot 2H_2O$ is a white, crystalline powder with molecular weight of 372.26. At room temperature, 11.1 g $Na_2H_2Y \cdot 2H_2O$ can be dissolved in 100 ml water. EDTA standard solution can be prepared by indirect method, that is, appropriate amount of $Na_2H_2Y \cdot 2H_2O$ is dissolved directly in water. The solution is then shaken well, and stored in a rigid glass bottle. The exact concentration of EDTA can be standardized using ZnO or Zn as primary standard and EBT or xylenol orange (XO) as indicator.

3. Apparatus and Materials

Apparatus: burette (25 ml), conical flask (250 ml), volumetric flask (500 ml), beaker (50 ml).

Materials: EDTA disodium salt ($Na_2H_2Y \cdot 2H_2O$), ZnO primary standard, dilute hydrochloric acid solution, methyl red indicator, ammonia solution, $NH_3 \cdot H_2O$ - NH_4Cl buffer solution, Eriochrome Black T (EBT) indicator.

4. Procedures

4.1 Preparation of 0.05 mol/L EDTA standard solution

9.5 g of $Na_2H_2Y \cdot 2H_2O$ is weighed, and dissolved with water. The solution is then transferred to 500 ml volumetric flask, diluted to the mark with water, and shaked well. The prepared solution is transferred to a hard glass bottle for storage.

4.2 Standardization of 0.05 mol/L EDTA standard solution

Accurately weigh out approximately 0.12 g of ZnO which is previously dried to constant weight at 800 ℃. It is dissolved in 3 ml of dilute hydrochloric acid, followed by adding 25 ml of distilled water and 1 drop of methyl red indicator. Ammonia solution is then added dropwise until the solution turns yellowish. After adding 25 ml of distilled water, 10 ml of $NH_3 \cdot H_2O$ - NH_4Cl buffer solution, and 2 drops of EBT indicator, the solution is titrated with EDTA solution until it changes from purplish red to pure blue.

The formula is as follows:

$$C_{EDTA} = \frac{W_{ZnO} \times 1000}{M_{ZnO} V_{EDTA}}$$

$$M_{ZnO} = 81.38$$

5. Notes

5.1　The dissolution of $Na_2H_2Y \cdot 2H_2O$ in water is slow, so constantly stirring or heating is usually used to accelerate the dissolution.

5.2　The prepared EDTA solution should be stored in a rigid glass bottle; otherwise, EDTA will react with the metal ions of the bottle, thereby affecting the concentration of EDTA.

5.3　The titration process should not be too fast. In particular, the titrant should be added dropwise and constantly shaken when nearing end point of titration.

6. Questions

6.1　What is the role of $NH_3 \cdot H_2O$ - NH_4Cl buffer solution?

6.2　Why do we need to add methyl red indicator in the experiment step and then add ammonia solution until the solution changes to a slight yellow?

实验八　EDTA 对铅、铋混合溶液的连续滴定

一、实验目的

1. 掌握控制溶液的酸度实现分步滴定的原理和方法。
2. 了解二甲酚橙指示剂终点的判断方法。

二、实验原理

如果溶液中存在两种或两种以上离子时，他们与 EDTA 的络合常数差别较大，即 $\Delta \lg K \geqslant 5$ 时，在没有其他配位剂的情况下，可通过控制溶液的酸度，使得只有 M 离子可以与 EDTA 形成稳定的络合物，而 N 离子不干扰滴定，从而实现两种离子的分步滴定。

Pb^{2+} 和 Bi^{3+} 都可以与 EDTA 反应形成稳定的络合物，它们的 $\lg K$ 值分别为 18.0 和 27.9。由于两者的 $\Delta \lg K$ 符合分步滴定的要求，他们的混合溶液就可以利用控制溶液酸度，实现 Bi^{3+} 和 Pb^{2+} 的连续滴定，分别测定它们在溶液中的含量。

二甲酚橙为红棕色结晶性粉末，易溶于水，不溶于无水乙醇。二甲酚橙作为指示剂常配成 0.2%的水溶液使用，pH＞6 时，呈现红色；pH＜6 时，呈现黄色。二甲酚橙与金属离子形成的配合物都是红紫色，因此它只适用于在 pH＜6 的酸性溶液中。二甲酚橙在 pH≈1 和 pH＝5～6 时可分别与 Bi^{3+} 和 Pb^{2+} 离子形成紫红色络合物。因此可以在溶液 pH≈1 时，用 EDTA 滴定 Bi^{3+}，然后在 pH＝5～6 时滴定 Pb^{2+}，终点颜色变化极为明显，均由紫红色突变为亮黄色。

三、仪器和材料

仪器　酸式滴定管（50 ml），锥形瓶（250 ml），移液管（25 ml），量筒（10 ml）。

材料　EDTA 标准溶液（0.01 mol/L），HNO_3 溶液（0.1 mol/L）；NaOH 溶液（0.1 mol/L），20%六亚甲基四胺，0.2%二甲酚橙水溶液，Bi^{3+}、Pb^{2+}混合溶液（约 0.01 mol/L），精密 pH（0.5～5）试纸。

四、实验步骤

1. EDTA 滴定 Bi^{3+}　准确移取 Bi^{3+} 和 Pb^{2+} 的混合液 25 ml 于 250 ml 锥形瓶中，用 0.1 mol/L 的 NaOH 溶液和 0.1 mol/L 的 HNO_3 溶液调节溶液的酸度至 pH≈1，再加入 10 ml 0.1 mol/L HNO_3 和 1～2 滴二甲酚橙指示剂，用 EDTA 标准溶液滴定至溶液由紫红色变为亮黄色，即为终点。记下消耗的 EDTA 标准溶液的体积。

2. EDTA 滴定 Pb^{2+}　在上述溶液中加入 20%六亚甲基四胺至溶液出现紫红色后，再加入 5 ml，继续用 EDTA 标准溶液滴定至溶液由紫红色突变为亮黄色，即为终点。记下消耗的 EDTA 标准溶液的体积。

根据两次滴定消耗的 EDTA 标准溶液的体积和 EDTA 标准溶液的浓度，可分别计算溶液中 Bi^{3+} 和 Pb^{2+} 的含量。

五、注意事项

调节溶液 pH≈1 时，溶液 pH 采用精密 pH 试纸测定，此时应尽量减少样品的取用量，以免因溶液损失引入较大的误差。

六、思考

同一份试液滴定两种离子的顺序是否可以改变？为什么？

Experiment 8　Continuous Titration of Pb^{2+} and Bi^{3+} Mixed Solution by EDTA

1. Objective

1.1　Master the principle and method of step‑by‑step titration by controlling acidity of the solution.

1.2　Understand the judgement of the end point by xylenol orange (XO) indicator.

2. Principle

If there are two or more ions in the solution, and their complexing constant with EDTA differ greatly, that is, $\Delta lgK \geqslant 5$, these ions can be titrated stepwise by controlling the acidity of the solution. That is, M ion can be titrated with EDTA, while the N ion does not interfere with the titration.

Both Pb^{2+} and Bi^{3+} can react with EDTA to form stable complexes with lgK values of 18.0 and 27.9, respectively. Because the ΔlgK meets the requirements of stepwise titration, their mixed solution can be titrated stepwise to respectively determine their content by controlling the acidity of the solution.

Xylenol orange (XO) is reddish brown crystalline powder, soluble in water, and insoluble in ethanol. Xylenol orange is often formulated into a 0.2% aqueous solution as an indicator, with the color of solution red when pH>6, and yellow when pH<6. The color of complex of xylenol orange and metal ions is purple, so xylenol orange is only suitable for acidic solution of pH<6. Xylenol orange can form a purple complex with Bi^{3+} and Pb^{2+} ions at pH≈1 and pH=5~6, respectively. Therefore, it is possible to titrate Bi^{3+} with EDTA at pH≈1, and then titrate Pb^{2+} with pH=5~6. The color change at the end point is extremely obvious, that is, the solution changes from red to bright yellow.

3. Apparatus and Materials

Apparatus: acidu burette (50 ml), conical flask (250 ml), pipette (25 ml), cylinder (10 ml).

Materials: EDTA standard solution (0.01 mol/L), HNO_3 solution (0.1 mol/L), NaOH solution (0.1 mol/L), 20% hexamethylene tetramine, 0.2% xylenol orange aqueous solution, precision pH (0.5~5) test paper.

4. Procedures

4.1　Titration of Bi³⁺

Pipette 25 ml mixture of Bi^{3+} and Pb^{2+} into 250 ml conical flask. 0.1 mol/L NaOH solution and 0.1 mol/L HNO_3 solution are then used to adjust the acidity of the solution to pH≈1. After adding 10 ml 0.1 mol/L HNO_3 and 1~2 drops of xylenol orange indicator, the solution is titrated with EDTA standard solution until the color of the solution changes from purple to bright yellow. Make a note of the volume of EDTA standard solution consumed.

4.2　Titration of Pb²⁺

Adding 20% hexamethylenetetramine to the above solution until purple color appears in the solution, and then adds 5 ml more. The solution is continued to titrate with EDTA standard solution until the color changes from purple to bright yellow, which is the end point. Make a note of the volume of EDTA standard solution consumed.

The contents of Bi^{3+} and Pb^{2+} in the solution can be calculated respectively based on the volume of EDTA standard solution consumed and the concentration of EDTA standard solution.

5. Notes

In the experimental step of adjusting acidity to pH≈1, the pH of the solution is measured using a precision pH test paper, so the amount of sample taken should minimize to avoid introducing large errors due to sample loss.

6. Questions

Whether the order of the two ions titration can be changed? Why?

实验九　EDTA 标准溶液的标定及自来水总硬度的测定

一、实验目的

1. 掌握 EDTA 标准溶液的配制和标定。
2. 掌握水硬度测定的原理和方法。
3. 了解配位滴定法的原理和应用。

二、实验原理

钙和镁是自来水中的主要金属离子，此外还含有微量的 Fe^{3+}、Al^{3+}、Cu^{2+}、Zn^{2+}、Pb^{2+} 等。世界各国有不同表示水硬度的方法，在中国，用相当于 CaO 量的 Ca^{2+}、Mg^{2+} 的数量代表水的总硬度。1° 是指在 1 L 水中含有 10 mg CaO，即 1° = 10 mg CaO/L。此外，水硬度还包括钙镁硬度，是分别测定钙和镁的浓度。

水质可以根据水的硬度分类。极软水为 0°～4°，软水为 4°～8°，中硬水为 8°～16°，硬水为 16°～30°，极硬水大于 30°。自来水的总硬度一般要小于 25°。

本实验采用配位滴定法测定自来水的总硬度，在 pH = 10 的氨性缓冲溶液中，以铬黑 T 作指示剂，以三乙醇胺、硫化钠掩蔽水样中存有 Fe^{3+}、Al^{3+}、Cu^{2+}、Zn^{2+}、Pb^{2+} 等微量杂质离子，用 EDTA 标准溶液直接滴定水中的 Ca^{2+}、Mg^{2+} 含量。计算水的总硬度可用下面的公式：

$$水的总硬度 = \frac{C_{EDTA} \cdot V_{EDTA} \cdot M_{CaO}}{V_{水} \cdot 10} \times 1000$$

三、仪器与材料

仪器　分析天平，滴定管（50 ml），锥形瓶（250 ml），容量瓶（250 ml），烧杯（100 ml），移液管（25 ml），量筒（50 ml）。

材料　EDTA 二钠盐，$CaCO_3$（基准），HCl（1:1），三乙醇胺（20%），Na_2S（2%），铬黑 T 指示剂，氨性缓冲溶液（pH = 10）。

四、试验步骤

1. $CaCO_3$ 标准溶液的配制　在称量瓶中用减量法精确称取 0.3～0.4 g $CaCO_3$，倒入 250 ml 烧杯中，加少许水润湿，盖上表面皿，缓慢滴入约 20 ml HCl（1:1）溶液，使 $CaCO_3$ 完全溶解。然后将 $CaCO_3$ 溶液置于 250 ml 容量瓶中，用水定容，摇匀。

2. EDTA 溶液（0.01 mol/L）的配制及标定　称取 1.0 g EDTA 二钠盐置于烧杯中，加 100 ml 水，微微加热搅拌使其完全溶解，冷却后稀释至 250 ml，转入试剂瓶中待标定。

用移液管移取 25 ml $CaCO_3$ 标液于 250 ml 锥形瓶，加 20 ml 氨性缓冲溶液和少许铬黑

T 指示剂，用 EDTA 溶液滴定至由紫红色变为蓝绿色，即为终点，记下所用体积，平行测定三份，计算 EDTA 标准溶液的浓度。

3. 水样总硬度的测定 用移液管移取 25 ml 自来水水样于 250 ml 锥形瓶中，加 1.5 ml 三乙醇胺，2.5 ml 氨性缓冲液，2～3 滴 Na_2S，2～3 滴铬黑 T 指示剂，用 EDTA 溶液滴定至溶液由紫红色变为蓝绿色，即为终点，记下所用体积，平行测定三份，计算水的总硬度。

五、注意事项

EDTA 标准溶液配制时可加入少量的镁盐,以提高终点变色的敏锐性。

六、思考

1. 测定水的总硬度有何实际意义？
2. 如要分别测定出钙、镁含量应如何进行？

Experiment 9　EDTA Solution Calibration and Determination of Tap Water Hardness

1. Objective

1.1　Master the principle and the method of water hardness determination.

1.2　Master EDTA solution preparation and calibration.

1.3　Learn the theory and application of complexometric titration.

2. Principle

Calcium and magnesium are the main metal ions in tap water. It also contains trace amounts of Fe^{3+}, Al^{3+}, Cu^{2+}, Pb^{2+}, Zn^{2+}, etc. Different countries in the world have different ways of expressing water hardness, In China, the amount of Ca^{2+}, Mg^{2+} ions equivalent to the amount of CaO is used to represent the total hardness of water. $1°$ means water containing 10 mg CaO in one liter. That is $1° = 10$ mg CaO/L. In addition，the water hardness also includes calcium magnesium hardness, it's measured by concentration of calcium and magnesium respectively.

The water quality can be classified according to the hardness of the water. Very soft water is $0°$ to $4°$, soft water to be $4°$ and $8°$, medium hard water to be $8°$ to $16°$, hard water to be $16°$ to $30°$, very hard water to be more than $30°$. The total hardness of tap water generally is less than $25°$.

In this study, EDTA complexometric titration can be used to determine total water hardness. In pH10 ammonia buffer solution, with eriochrome black T as indicator, with triethanolamine and Na_2S masking Fe^{3+}, Al^{3+}, Cu^{2+}, Pb^{2+}, Zn^{2+} and other ions, total water hardness can be directly measured by EDTA standard solution titration.

The following formula can be used to calculate the hardness of water.

$$\text{total water hardness} = \frac{C_{EDTA} \cdot V_{EDTA} \cdot M_{CaO}}{V_{water} \cdot 10} \times 1000$$

$$M_{CaO} = 56$$

3. Apparatus and Materials

Apparatus: analytical balance, burette (50 ml), conical flask (250 ml), volumetric flask(250 ml), beaker (100 ml), graduated pipette (25 ml), cylinder (50 ml).

Materials: standard $CaCO_3$, EDTA‐2Na, HCl, triethanolamine (20%), Na_2S (2%), Eriochrome Black T, ammonia buffer solution (pH = 10).

4. Procedures

4.1 Preparation of CaCO₃ standard solution

Accurately weigh 0.3~0.4 g $CaCO_3$ in a weighing bottle with decrement method, poured into 250 ml beaker, add a little water until wetting, cover the surface of dish, drop slowly about 20 ml HCl(1:1) solution, so that $CaCO_3$ is completely dissolved. Then transfer the $CaCO_3$ solution in 250 ml volumetric flask and set to the mark with water, shake well.

4.2 0.01 mol / L EDTA standard solution for calibration

Weigh 1.0 g EDTA-2Na into a beaker, add 100 ml of water, slightly heat and stir to dissolve completely, turn into a reagent bottle after cooling, dilute to 250 ml, and shake well for calibrating.

Pipet 25 ml $CaCO_3$ standard solution into a 250 ml conical flask, add 20 ml ammonia buffer solution, 3 drops of eriochrome black T indicator, immediately titrate with EDTA standard solution, when the solution stabilizes by a wine red to blue purple and then just end shall be. Note reading, measure three times in parallel; calculate the concentration of EDTA solution.

4.3 Determination of water hardness

Measure 25 ml of tap water with graduated cylinder into 250 ml conical flask, add 1.5 ml of triethanolamine and 10 ml of ammonia buffer solution, 2~3 drops of Na_2S and 2~3 drops of eriochrome black T indicator, immediately titrate with EDTA standard solution. When the solution changes to blue purple, it is the end point and then titration volume is recorded. Measure three times in parallel, calculate the total water hardness.

5. Notes

A little magnesium salt can be added into the preparation of EDTA standard solution to improve the sensitivity of terminal discoloration.

6. Questions

6.1　Practical significance of the determination of total hardness of water.

6.2　How to determine the contents of calcium and magnesium respectively?

实验十　0.1 mol/L Na₂S₂O₃标准溶液的配制和标定

一、实验目的

1. 掌握 $Na_2S_2O_3$ 溶液的配制方法及配制注意事项。
2. 掌握采用基准物质 $K_2Cr_2O_7$ 标定 $Na_2S_2O_3$ 标准溶液的方法。

二、实验原理

结晶硫代硫酸钠（$Na_2S_2O_3 \cdot 5H_2O$）常易风化或潮解，并含有少量杂质。因此，$Na_2S_2O_3$ 标准溶液需采用间接法配制。

$Na_2S_2O_3$ 溶液不稳定，易分解。水中的 CO_2、O_2、细菌以及光照都能使其分解，故配制 $Na_2S_2O_3$ 溶液时，常采用新煮沸放冷的蒸馏水，以除去水中的 CO_2 和 O_2 并杀死细菌；加入少量 Na_2CO_3 使溶液呈弱碱性（pH9～10），以抑制 $Na_2S_2O_3$ 的分解和细菌的生长；溶液贮存于棕色瓶中，在暗处放置7～10天，待浓度稳定后进行标定。

标定 $Na_2S_2O_3$ 溶液可用 KIO_3、$K_2Cr_2O_7$、$KBrO_3$ 等基准物质，其中 $K_2Cr_2O_7$ 最为常用。在酸性溶液中，一定量的 $K_2Cr_2O_7$ 与过量的 KI 作用置换出 I_2，以淀粉作指示剂，再用 $Na_2S_2O_3$ 溶液滴定，其反应如下：

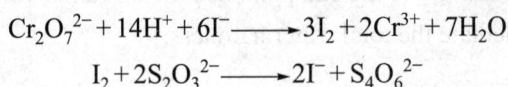

$$Cr_2O_7^{2-} + 14H^+ + 6I^- \longrightarrow 3I_2 + 2Cr^{3+} + 7H_2O$$

$$I_2 + 2S_2O_3^{2-} \longrightarrow 2I^- + S_4O_6^{2-}$$

$Cr_2O_7^{2-}$ 与 I^- 的反应速度较慢，为了加快反应速度，可控制溶液酸度 0.5 mol/L 左右为宜，同时加入过量的 KI，并在暗处放置一定时间。但在滴定前需将溶液稀释，既可降低酸度从而防止 $Na_2S_2O_3$ 分解，又可降低 Cr^{3+} 的浓度，使其亮绿色变浅，便于观察终点。淀粉指示剂应在近终点时加入，当溶液蓝色消失即为终点。

三、仪器和材料

仪器　酸式滴定管（25 ml），烧杯（100 ml），碘量瓶（250 ml），量筒（10 ml、100 ml），移液管（20 ml），试剂瓶（1000 ml）。

材料　$Na_2S_2O_3 \cdot 5H_2O$（分析纯），KI（分析纯），HCl 溶液（1:2），$K_2Cr_2O_7$（基准试剂），0.5%淀粉溶液。

四、实验步骤

1. 0.1 mol/L Na₂S₂O₃ 标准溶液的配制　在 1000 ml 含有 0.2 g Na_2CO_3 的新煮沸放冷的蒸馏水中加入 $Na_2S_2O_3 \cdot 5H_2O$ 26 g，使完全溶解，放置 2 周后再标定。

2. 0.1 mol/L Na₂S₂O₃ 标准溶液的标定　准确称量基准物质 $K_2Cr_2O_7$ 0.10～0.12 g 于250 ml 碘量瓶中，加 25 ml 蒸馏水溶解。加入 2 g KI，轻轻振摇直至全部溶解。加入 25 ml

水和 5 ml HCl 溶液（1:2），盖上瓶塞，同时旋摇使溶液混匀，水封，在暗处放置 10 min。加蒸馏水 50 ml 稀释，用 $Na_2S_2O_3$ 溶液滴定至近终点，加淀粉指示液 2 ml，继续滴定至蓝色消失而显亮绿色，即为终点。重复标定 2 次，相对偏差不能超过 0.2%。按下式计算 $Na_2S_2O_3$ 溶液的浓度。

$$C_{Na_2S_2O_3} = \frac{6W_{K_2Cr_2O_7}}{V_{Na_2S_2O_3} \times M_{K_2Cr_2O_7} / 1000}$$

$$M_{K_2Cr_2O_7} = 294.18$$

五、注意事项

1. $K_2Cr_2O_7$ 与 KI 反应较慢，在稀溶液中更慢，故在加水稀释前，应放置 10 min，使反应完全。

2. 滴定前，溶液要加水稀释。

3. 酸度影响滴定。

4. KI 要过量，但浓度不能超过 2%~4%，因为 I⁻ 浓度太高，淀粉指示剂颜色转变不灵敏。

5. 由于空气中氧气的氧化会使溶液缓慢回蓝，但不影响结果。如果回蓝迅速，说明 $K_2Cr_2O_7$ 与 KI 反应不完全。

六、思考

1. 配制 $Na_2S_2O_3$ 溶液时需要注意哪些问题？

2. 在滴定前为什么要将溶液在暗处放置 10 min？为什么要加水稀释后再滴定？

3. 如何防止 I_2 挥发和空气氧化 I⁻？

4. 为什么在近终点加入淀粉指示剂？过早加入会出现什么现象？

Experiment 10　Preparation and Standardization of 0.1 mol/L Sodium Thiosulfate Standard Solution

1. Objective

1.1　Master the preparation of sodium thiosulfate standard solution and the notes.

1.2　Master the method of standardization of sodium thiosulfate with the primary standard $K_2Cr_2O_7$.

2. Principle

Crystalline sodium thiosulfate ($Na_2S_2O_3 \cdot 5H_2O$) is easily weathered or deliquescent and contains a small amount of impurities. Therefore, the $Na_2S_2O_3$ standard solution should be prepared by indirect method.

Sodium thiosulfate solution is unstable and easy to be decomposed. It can be decomposed by CO_2, O_2, bacteria in water and sunlight, so when preparing $Na_2S_2O_3$ solution, the cold, recently boiled distilled water is often used to remove CO_2 and O_2 and kill bacteria. A small amount of Na_2CO_3 is added to the solution in order to inhibit the decomposition of $Na_2S_2O_3$ and the growth of bacteria, the solution is stored in a brown bottle and placed in the dark for 7~10 days, it will be standardized after the concentration is stable.

Standardization of $Na_2S_2O_3$ can use KIO_3、$K_2Cr_2O_7$ and $KBrO_3$ as the primary standard substance. $K_2Cr_2O_7$ is the commonly used. In acid solution, a certain amount of $K_2Cr_2O_7$ react with excessive KI to form I_2, the starch solution is used as an indicator, and $Na_2S_2O_3$ solution is used as titrating solution. The titration reaction can be written as follows:

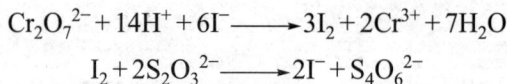

$$Cr_2O_7^{2-} + 14H^+ + 6I^- \longrightarrow 3I_2 + 2Cr^{3+} + 7H_2O$$

$$I_2 + 2S_2O_3^{2-} \longrightarrow 2I^- + S_4O_6^{2-}$$

The reaction rate of $Cr_2O_7^{2-}$ and I^- is relatively slow. In order to accelerate the reaction rate, it is appropriate to control the acidity of the solution about 0.5 mol/L, at the same time adding excessive KI, and keeping it in the dark for a certain time. However, the solution should be diluted before titration, which can not only lower the acidity to prevent $Na_2S_2O_3$ from decomposing, but also lower the concentration of Cr^{3+}, making it light green and easy to observe the end point. Starch indicator must be added just before the end point is reached, when the blue of solution disappears, it will be the end point.

3. Apparatus and Materials

Apparatus: acid burette (25 ml), beaker (100 ml), iodine flask (250 ml), cylinder (10 ml、100 ml), pipette (20 ml), reagent bottle (1000 ml).

Materials: $Na_2S_2O_3 \cdot 5H_2O$ (A.R)，KI (A.R)，HCl Solution (1:2)，$K_2Cr_2O_7$ (primary reagent)，0.5% starch solution.

4. Procedures

4.1　Preparation of 0.1 mol/L $Na_2S_2O_3$ standard solution

Place 26 g of $Na_2S_2O_3 \cdot 5H_2O$ in 1000 ml of cold, recently boiled distilled water containing 0.2 g of mild alkali Na_2CO_3. Dissolve it completely, and allow to stand for fortnight before standardization.

4.2　Standardization of 0.1 mol/L $Na_2S_2O_3$ standard solution

Weigh out accurately 0.10~0.12 g of primary standard $K_2Cr_2O_7$ into 250 ml iodine flask. Dissolve in 25 ml of distilled water. Add 2 g of KI and shake gently until the salt dissolves. Add 25 ml of water and 5 ml of HCl solution (1:2), stopper it whilst gently rotate to mix the solution well, cover it with water, allow the solution to stand in dark for 10 minutes, and dilute with 50 ml of water. Titrate with $Na_2S_2O_3$ solution to near end point, then add 2 ml of starch solution, continue titration until the color of the solution change from greenish - blue to light green. That's the end point. Repeat twice as described above. Relative deviation of the results must be within 0.2%. Calculate the concentration of the sodium thiosulfate solution by the following formula.

$$C_{Na_2S_2O_3} = \frac{6W_{K_2Cr_2O_7}}{V_{Na_2S_2O_3} \times M_{K_2Cr_2O_7} / 1000}$$

$$M_{K_2Cr_2O_7} = 294.18$$

5. Notes

5.1　The reaction rate of $K_2Cr_2O_7$ and KI is relatively slow, especially in dilute solution. In order to make the reaction complete, the solution should be allowed to stand for 10 minutes before adding water

5.2　The dilution of solution should be made before the titration.

5.3　Acidity affects titration.

5.4　An excess of KI should be needed but it should not be more than 2%~4%. Because if the concentration iodine ion is too high, the color change of starch indicator will be not sensitive.

5.5　It is possible that the color of solution returns slowly to blue at the end point because of oxidation of oxygen in air. It doesn't affect the result of this experiment. If this returning occurs quickly, it shows that the reaction of $K_2Cr_2O_7$ with KI is not complete.

6. Questions

6.1   What problems should you pay attention to in the preparation of $Na_2S_2O_3$ solution?

6.2   It is necessary to allow the solution to stand in dark for 10 minutes and dilute it with water before the titration is made, why?

6.3   How to prevent I_2 from volatilizing and I^- being oxidized by air?

6.4   Why must starch solution be added just before the end point is reached? And what will happen if starch solution is too early added?

实验十一　碘量法测定维生素 C 的含量

一、实验目的

1. 了解用碘量法测定维生素 C 含量的原理。
2. 进一步熟悉电子天平的使用和滴定操作。

二、实验原理

氧化还原滴定法是利用氧化还原反应为基础的容量分析方法。几乎所有元素和许多有机化合物的含量，都能直接或间接地利用氧化还原法进行测定，因此它的应用范围极为广泛。根据所用氧化剂种类的不同，氧化还原法可以分成高锰酸钾法、重铬酸钾法、碘量法和溴酸钾法等。I_2/I^- 电对的标准电极电势为 0.535 V，因此 I_2 是较弱的氧化剂，只能与较强的还原剂作用；而 I^- 是中等强度的还原剂，能与许多强氧化剂及一般中等强度的氧化剂作用。由于这些特点，碘量法在生产实践中获得了广泛的应用。

维生素 C 又名抗坏血酸，分子式为 $C_6H_8O_6$，通常用于防治坏血病及各种慢性传染病的辅助治疗。市售维生素 C 片含淀粉等添加剂。由于维生素 C 分子中的烯二醇基具有较强的还原性，故能被 I_2 定量地氧化成二酮基。

维生素 C 的半反应：

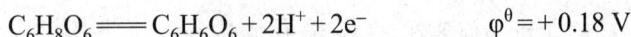

$$C_6H_8O_6 \Longrightarrow C_6H_6O_6 + 2H^+ + 2e^- \qquad\qquad \varphi^\theta = +0.18\ V$$

1 mol 维生素 C 与 1 mol I_2 定量反应，维生素 C 的摩尔质量为 176.12 g/mol。

维生素 C 的还原性很强，在空气中极易被氧化，尤其在碱性介质中更甚，所以测定时加入 HAc 使溶液呈弱酸性，减少维生素 C 的副反应，避免引起实验误差。

I_2 溶液的浓度可以由已知浓度的 $Na_2S_2O_3$ 标准溶液滴定，以淀粉溶液为指示剂，滴定至蓝色刚好消失即为终点，它们之间发生如下反应：

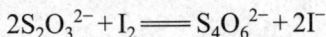

$$2S_2O_3^{2-} + I_2 \Longrightarrow S_4O_6^{2-} + 2I^-$$

根据以上反应，可计算出药片中维生素 C 的含量：

$$W_{C_6H_8O_6}(\%) = \frac{C_{I_2} V_{I_2} M_{C_6H_8O_6}}{m_{C_6H_8O_6}} \times 100\%$$

式中：C_{I_2}，I_2 溶液的浓度；V_{I_2}，滴定时所用 I_2 溶液的体积；$M_{C_6H_8O_6}$，维生素 C 的摩尔质量；$m_{C_6H_8O_6}$，称取的维生素 C 的质量。

三、仪器和材料

仪器　研钵，容量瓶（100 ml），锥形瓶（250 ml），酸式滴定管（25 ml），烧杯（500 ml），量筒（100 ml、50 ml、10 ml）、移液管（25 ml）、电子天平。

材料 维生素 C 片，新煮沸过的冷蒸馏水，$Na_2S_2O_3$ 标准溶液，淀粉溶液（0.5%），HAc 溶液（0.02 mol/L），I_2 溶液。

四、实验步骤

1. I_2 溶液的标定 准确吸取 $Na_2S_2O_3$ 标准溶液 25.00 ml 三份，分别置于 250 ml 锥形瓶中，加水 50 ml，淀粉溶液 2 ml，用 I_2 溶液滴定成稳定的蓝色，半分钟内显色不褪色即为终点。然后计算 I_2 溶液的浓度，相对偏差不超过 ±0.5%。

2. 维生素 C 片的含量测定

（1）将维生素 C 片用研钵研成粉末，用电子天平减重称量维生素 C 三份，分别放入三个 100 ml 的量瓶中，每份 0.2～0.3 g。

（2）在量瓶中，加入新煮沸过的冷蒸馏水适量，0.02 mol/L HAc 溶液 1 ml，振摇使维生素 C 溶解并稀释至刻度，摇匀，迅速滤过，取续滤液 50 ml，加淀粉溶液 2 ml，立即用 I_2 溶液滴定，至呈现稳定的蓝色，即为终点。

（3）按同样方法滴定另两份

（4）计算维生素 C 的含量

五、注意事项

1. 使用滴定管前要进行试漏。
2. 滴定剩余的碘滴定液要放回回收瓶。

六、思考

1. 测定维生素 C 的含量为何要在 HAc 介质中进行？
2. 溶解维生素 C 试样，为何要用新煮沸过的冷蒸馏水？
3. 本实验产生误差的原因主要有哪些？

Experiment 11　Vitamin C Determination by Iodine Titration

1. Objective

1.1　To understand the principle of Vitamin C determination using iodine method.

1.2　Be familiar with electronic balance and titration operation.

2. Principle

Redox titration is a volumetry made on the basis of oxidation-reduction reaction. Redox titration is widely used in analysis. Almost all of elements and many organic compounds can be determined by redox titration. Potassium permanganate, iodine, potassium dichromate and potassium bromate are commonly used oxidant.

The standard electrode potentials of I_2/I^- is 0.535 V. As a weak oxidant, I_2 can only act with strong reductant. I^- has a stronger reducing potential, it can act with not only strong oxidant but also medium oxidants. Thus, iodine method has been widely used in industry.

Vitamin C (L-ascorbic acid, $C_6H_8O_6$) is an antioxidant that is essential for human nutrition. It is used for the treatment of prevention of scurvy and various chronic infectious diseases. Generally, Vitamin C tablets contain starch and other additives. As an enediol-containing compound, Vitamin C can quantitatively undergo a rapid redox reaction with I_2, and then it is converted to diketone.

The half-reaction of Vitamin C is as follow:

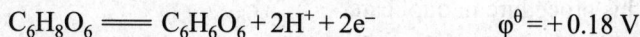

$$C_6H_8O_6 \rightleftharpoons C_6H_6O_6 + 2H^+ + 2e^- \qquad \varphi^\theta = +0.18 \text{ V}$$

1 mol Vitamin C quantitatively acts with 1 mol I_2. The molecular weight of Vitamin C is 176.12 g/mol.

As Vitamin C is a strong reductant, it is easy to be oxidized in the air or alkaline medium. Acetic acid should be added to avoid the side reaction of Vitamin C.

Use standard $Na_2S_2O_3$ solution as titrant to titrate I_2 solution, to calculate the concentration of I_2 solution. At the end point, I_2 will be exhausted and the blue color will disappear:

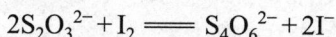

$$2S_2O_3^{2-} + I_2 \rightleftharpoons S_4O_6^{2-} + 2I^-$$

According to the reaction described above, we can calculate the concentration of Vitamin C in tablets.

$$W_{C_6H_8O_6}(\%) = \frac{C_{I_2} V_{I_2} M_{C_6H_8O_6}}{m_{C_6H_8O_6}} \times 100\%$$

Note: C_{I_2} —concentration of I_2 solution;

V_{I_2} —volume of I_2 solution used;

$M_{C_6H_8O_6}$ —molecular weight of Vitamin C;

$m_{C_6H_8O_6}$ —Vitamin C tablets weight

3. Apparatus and Materials

Apparatus: volumetric flask (100 ml), mortar, conical flask (250 ml), acid buret (25 ml), beaker (500 ml), cylinder (100 ml, 50 ml and 10 ml), pipette (25 ml) and electronic balance.

Materials: vitamin C tablets, fresh distilled water cold, $Na_2S_2O_3$ standard solution, 0.5% starch solution, 0.02 mol/L acetic acid, I_2 solution.

4. Procedures

4.1 Standardization of I_2 solution

Add 25 ml $Na_2S_2O_3$ standard solutions to 250 ml conical flask in triplicate, then add 50 ml distilled water and 2 ml 0.5% starch solution, respectively. Use I_2 solution to titrate and from the blue color. Keep blue color and it is the endpoint of the titration. Next, calculate the concentration of I_2 solution. The relative error should not exceed $\pm 0.5\%$.

4.2 Determination of Vitamin C

4.2.1   Crush Vitamin C tablets with mortar, weight powder $0.2\sim0.3$ g using balance in triplicate.

4.2.2   Appropriate amount of fresh cold distilled water, 1 ml of 0.02 mol/L acetic acid and weighed Vitamin C powder mix well in 100 ml volumetric flask. Dissolve the Vitamin C and dilute to the final volume (100 ml). Then this solution is filtrated. Use I_2 solution to titrate 50 ml filtrate, immediately. At the equivalence point, any I_2 produced thereafter will react with starch indicator to produce a blue color to indicate the end point.

4.2.3   Repeat this procedure in duplicate.

4.2.4   Calculate the concentration of Vitamin C.

5. Cautions

5.1   Leakage test is needed before using the buret.

5.2   Withdraw the remaining I_2 after titrating.

6. Questions

6.1   Why Vitamin C must be determined in acetic acid medium?

6.2   Why Vitamin C must be dissolved in fresh cold distilled water?

6.3   What cause the major error of this experiment?

实验十二　碘量法测定葡萄糖的含量

一、实验目的

1. 掌握间接碘量法测定葡萄糖含量的原理和方法。
2. 学习间接碘量法中剩余回滴法的操作。
3. 进行空白实验的练习。

二、实验原理

碘可与氢氧化钠作用生成次碘酸钠，次碘酸钠能定量地将葡糖糖氧化成葡萄糖酸盐，未与葡萄糖反应的 NaIO 在碱性溶液中转变成 $NaIO_3$ 和 NaI。当酸化溶液时，$NaIO_3$ 又恢复成 I_2，析出的 I_2，即剩余的 I_2，用 $Na_2S_2O_3$ 标准溶液滴定剩余的 I_2 进而计算出葡萄糖的含量。反应方程式如下：

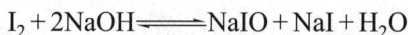

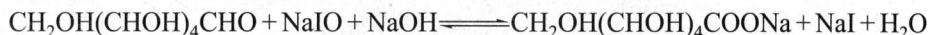

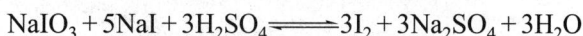

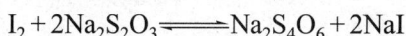

$$I_2 + 2NaOH \Longrightarrow NaIO + NaI + H_2O$$

$$CH_2OH(CHOH)_4CHO + NaIO + NaOH \Longrightarrow CH_2OH(CHOH)_4COONa + NaI + H_2O$$

$$3NaIO \Longrightarrow NaIO_3 + 2NaI$$

$$NaIO_3 + 5NaI + 3H_2SO_4 \Longrightarrow 3I_2 + 3Na_2SO_4 + 3H_2O$$

$$I_2 + 2Na_2S_2O_3 \Longrightarrow Na_2S_4O_6 + 2NaI$$

三、仪器和材料

仪器　碱式滴定管（25 ml），碘量瓶（250 ml），量筒（10 ml，100 ml），移液管（25 ml）。

材料　葡萄糖（药用），碘标准溶液（0.05 mol/L），$Na_2S_2O_3$ 标准溶液（0.1 mol/L），0.1 mol/L NaOH 溶液，0.5 mol/L H_2SO_4 溶液，0.5%淀粉溶液。

四、实验步骤

取样品约 0.1 g，精密称定，置 250 ml 碘量瓶中，加蒸馏水 30 ml 使溶解。加入 0.05 mol/L I_2 溶液 25.00 ml，在不断摇动下缓慢滴加 0.1 mol/L NaOH 溶液 40 ml，直至溶液呈浅黄色。密塞，水封，暗处放置 10 min。加入 0.5 mol/L H_2SO_4 溶液 6 ml，摇匀，用 $Na_2S_2O_3$ 标准溶液（0.1 mol/L）回滴剩余的 I_2。近终点时加入淀粉指示液 2 ml，继续滴定至溶液蓝色消失，即为终点。同时做空白实验。由获得的数据，按下式计算葡萄糖的含量：

$$葡萄糖\% = \frac{C_{Na_2S_2O_3} \left[V_0 - V_{(样品)} \right]}{W_{葡萄糖}} \times \frac{M_{C_6H_{12}O_6 \cdot H_2O}}{2 \times 1000} \times 100\%$$

$$M_{C_6H_{12}O_6 \cdot H_2O} = 198.2$$

五、注意事项

滴加 NaOH 溶液时要缓慢滴加，否则过量的 NaIO 来不及与葡萄糖作用，本身发生歧化反应，生成不与葡萄糖作用的 $NaIO_3$ 而导致葡萄糖氧化不完全，使结果偏低。

六、思考

1. 本实验中如何判断滴定终点与近终点？
2. 葡萄糖与碘（I_2）化学反应的摩尔比是多少？

Experiment 12 Determination of Glucose by Iodimetry

1. Objective

1.1 Master the principle and method for the determination of glucose by indirect iodimetry.

1.2 Learn the operation of reisdue titration in indirect iodometry.

1.3 Practise the blank test.

2. Principle

Iodine can react with sodium hydroxide to form sodium hypoiodate. Sodium hypoiodate can quantitatively oxidize glucose to gluconate, and the NaIO which does not react with glucose is transformed into $NaIO_3$ and NaI in alkaline solution. When the solution is acidified, $NaIO_3$ is back into I_2. The precipitating I_2, namely, the residual I_2, can be titrated with $Na_2S_2O_3$ standard solution to calculate the content of glucose. The titration reaction can be written as follows:

$$I_2 + 2NaOH \rightleftharpoons NaIO + NaI + H_2O$$
$$CH_2OH(CHOH)_4CHO + NaIO + NaOH \rightleftharpoons CH_2OH(CHOH)_4COONa + NaI + H_2O$$
$$3NaIO \rightleftharpoons NaIO_3 + 2NaI$$
$$NaIO_3 + 5NaI + 3H_2SO_4 \rightleftharpoons 3I_2 + 3Na_2SO_4 + 3H_2O$$
$$I_2 + 2Na_2S_2O_3 \rightleftharpoons Na_2S_4O_6 + 2NaI$$

3. Apparatus and Materials

Apparatus: basic burette(25 ml), iodine flask (250 ml)，cylinder (10 ml, 100 ml)，pipette (25 ml).

Materials: medicinal glucose, iodine standard solution(0.05 mol/L), $Na_2S_2O_3$ standard solution (0.10 mol/L), 0.1 mol/L NaOH solution , 0.5 mol/L H_2SO_4 solution, 0.5% starch solution.

4. Procedures

Weigh out accurately 0.1 g of glucose into 250 ml iodine flask. Dissolve in 30 ml of distilled water. Add 25.00 ml iodine standard solution (0.05 mol/L), and drop 40 ml of 0.1 mol/L NaOH solution slowly with shaking constantly until the color of the solution is yellowish, stopper it, cover it with water, allow the solution to stand in dark for 10 minutes. Add 6 ml of 0.5 mol/L H_2SO_4 solution, shake the solution well, titrate the residual I_2 with $Na_2S_2O_3$ standard solution (0.10 mol/L) until the nearly endpoint, add 2 ml of starch solution and continue to titrate until the blue color of the solution disappear.

The blank test shoud be done simultaneously with sample test. From the data obtained, calculate the content of glucose as follows.

$$\text{Glucose\%} = \frac{C_{\text{Na}_2\text{S}_2\text{O}_3} \left[V_0 - V_{\text{sample}} \right]}{W_{\text{glucose}}} \times \frac{M_{\text{C}_6\text{H}_{12}\text{O}_6 \cdot \text{H}_2\text{O}}}{2 \times 1000} \times 100\%$$

$$M_{\text{C}_6\text{H}_{12}\text{O}_6 \cdot \text{H}_2\text{O}} = 198.2$$

5. Notes

Dropping speed of NaOH solution shouldn't be too fast, otherwise, there is no time for excessive NaIO to react with glucose. The disproportionation reaction will take place, generate $NaIO_3$, which can't react with glucose, leading the oxidation of glucose incompletely, making the result to the low side.

6. Questions

6.1　How to judge endpoint and nearly endpoint when I_2 is titrated by the $Na_2S_2O_3$?

6.2　What is the mole ratio of the glucose to I_2?

实验十三　0.02 mol/L 高锰酸钾标准溶液的配制与标定

一、实验目的

1. 掌握高锰酸钾溶液的配制与保存。
2. 掌握用草酸钠作为基准物质标定高锰酸钾溶液的原理、条件和方法。
3. 掌握使用自身指示剂判断滴定终点。

二、实验原理

在酸性溶液中高锰酸钾是一种强氧化剂，其电极反应方程式如下：

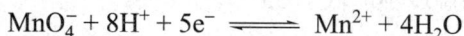

$$MnO_4^- + 8H^+ + 5e^- \rightleftharpoons Mn^{2+} + 4H_2O$$

滴定应该在硫酸中进行，一般来说溶液的酸度应该维持在 1~2 mol/L，市售的高锰酸钾一般含有杂质，如二氧化锰、氯化钠、硫酸盐、硝酸等。因而不能在配制标准溶液中直接使用。另外高锰酸钾的氧化能力很强，很容易与水中有机杂质、空气中的灰尘等还原物质反应。光照很容易分解，当配制时，溶液必须煮沸或用煮沸并冷却的蒸馏水溶解，并保存在棕色的试剂瓶中避光。高锰酸钾溶液通常可用草酸钠标定，反应方程式如下：

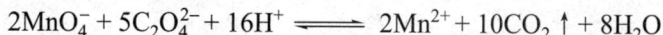

$$2MnO_4^- + 5C_2O_4^{2-} + 16H^+ \rightleftharpoons 2Mn^{2+} + 10CO_2\uparrow + 8H_2O$$

由于反应速度的很慢，所以必须加热。即使这样，反应仍然很慢，而且在开始滴定时，高锰酸钾的颜色不能很快的褪去，所以当开始滴定时，高锰酸钾必须逐滴加入，二价锰离子的产生会作为催化剂加速反应，所以滴定后期滴定速度可以提高一些。

由于高锰酸钾自身有颜色，所以可以通过高锰酸钾的颜色来指示终点。

三、仪器和材料

仪器　酸式滴定管（25 ml），锥形瓶（250 ml），烧杯（500 ml），量筒（10 ml，100 ml），棕色试剂瓶（500 ml），多孔玻璃烧结漏斗，电子分析天平。

材料　KMnO$_4$（A.R.），Na$_2$C$_2$O$_4$（基准物质），H$_2$SO$_4$。

四、实验步骤

1. 0.02 mol/L 高锰酸钾标准溶液的配制　用 500 ml 蒸馏水溶解 1.6 g 高锰酸钾于棕色瓶中，溶液避光放置 7~10 天，用多孔玻璃烧结漏斗过滤并保存在棕色试剂瓶中。

2. 高锰酸钾标准溶液的标定　精密称取 0.15 g 基准物质草酸钠，置 250 ml 的锥形瓶中，用 100 ml 蒸馏水和 5 ml 硫酸溶解，水浴加热到 75~85 ℃。不断振摇，用高锰酸钾溶液逐滴滴加，仅当前一滴粉红色褪色时再滴加，加入大约 15 ml 高锰酸钾溶液。在高锰酸钾褪色后，滴定继续进行，直至呈淡粉色，并持续 0.5 min，终点溶液的温度不应低于 55 ℃。高锰酸钾的摩尔浓度由如下公式计算：

$$C_{KMnO_4} = \frac{2 \times W_{Na_2C_2O_4}}{5 \times V_{KMnO_4} \times \dfrac{M_{Na_2C_2O_4}}{1000}}$$

$$M_{Na_2C_2O_4} = 134.0$$

五、注意事项

1. 市售的高锰酸钾不能直接配制成标准溶液，因为二氧化锰作为杂质存在，会加速高锰酸钾分解，二氧化锰可以通过过滤除去，注意不能用滤纸过滤。

2. 蒸馏水通常包含一些能还原高锰酸钾的杂质，所以蒸馏水在用之前需要煮沸。

3. 光照会加速高锰酸钾的分解，所以高锰酸钾溶液必须保存在棕色试剂瓶内，在暗处放置 7～10 天。

4. 反应很慢，因此开始滴定时不宜过快。

5. 滴定终点时溶液的温度不能低于 55 ℃。

六、思考

1. 为什么盐酸和硝酸不能用来控制酸度？

2. 当配制高锰酸钾溶液时，应该注意些什么？为什么？

Experiment 13 Preparation and Standardization of 0.02 mol/L Standard Potassium Permanganate Solution

1. Objective

1.1 Master the preparation and preservation of a potassium permanganate solution.

1.2 Master the principle, the condition and the method of standardization of $KMnO_4$ solution with the primary standard $Na_2C_2O_4$.

1.3 Master the use of self–indicator in the detection of endpoint.

2. Principle

Potassium permanganate ($KMnO_4$) is a vigorous oxidant in an acidic solution, and its electrode reaction as follow,

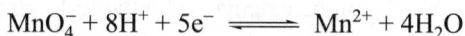

$$MnO_4^- + 8H^+ + 5e^- \rightleftharpoons Mn^{2+} + 4H_2O$$

The titration reaction should be carried out in sulfuric acid (H_2SO_4), in general, the acidity of the solution should be maintained at $1\sim2$ mol/L. $KMnO_4$ on sale usually contains impurities such as MnO_2, chloride, sulfate, nitrate and so on. Therefore, it cannot be used directly in the preparation of standard solution. Moreover, because the oxidization ability of $KMnO_4$ is strong, and it readily reacts with reductive substances such as organic impurities in water, ashes in air and so on, it easily decomposes when exposed to light. When it is prepared, its solution must be boiled or be dissolved with cold distilled water and then kept in brown reagent bottle in dark.

$KMnO_4$ solution generally can be standardized by sodium oxalate ($Na_2C_2O_4$). The reaction between $KMnO_4$ and $Na_2C_2O_4$ in an acidic solution is:

$$2MnO_4^- + 5C_2O_4^{2-} + 16H^+ \rightleftharpoons 2Mn^{2+} + 10CO_2 \uparrow + 8H_2O$$

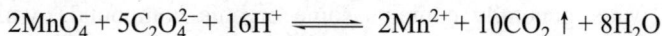

Heating up is necessary because the reaction is slow. Even if so, the reaction is still slow and the color of $KMnO_4$ can't fade rapidly at the beginning of the titration. So at the beginning of titration, the $KMnO_4$ solution must be titrated drop by drop for speed of reaction is very slow. But the reaction is accelerated once Mn^{2+}, catalyzer of the reaction, forms during the reaction, so titration speed may be increased slightly.

Because $KMnO_4$ solution itself has color, the endpoint can be indicated by the color of $KMnO_4$.

3. Apparatus and Materials

Apparatus: acid burette (25 ml), conical flask (250 ml), beaker (500 ml), cylinder (10 ml,

100 ml), brown bottle(500 ml), fine-porosity and sintered-glass funnel, electronic analytical balance.

Materials: $KMnO_4$ (A.R.), $Na_2C_2O_4$ (primary reagent), H_2SO_4.

4. Procedures

4.1 Preparation of 0.02 mol/L $KMnO_4$ standard solution

Dissolve about 1.6 g $KMnO_4$ in 500 ml of boiled distilled water in a brown bottle. The solution is allowed to stand in dark place for 7～10 days, filter through a fine-porosity, sintered–glass funnel and preserved in another brown bottle.

4.2 Standardization of $KMnO_4$ solution

Weigh out accurately about 0.15 g of primary standard $Na_2C_2O_4$ into 250 ml conical flask. Dissolve in 100 ml of water and 5 ml H_2SO_4. The solution is then heated to 75 ℃～85 ℃ using water bath. During continuous shaking, titrate it with $KMnO_4$ solution drop after drop only when the pink of the first drop fades, then add to about 15 ml $KMnO_4$ solution from a burette in it. After the color of $KMnO_4$ fades, titration will be continued until a pale pink color is observed and persists for 0.5 min. The temperature of the solution at the endpoint should not be less than 55 ℃. The concentration of $KMnO_4$ can be calculated by the following formula:

$$C_{KMnO_4} = \frac{2 \times W_{Na_2C_2O_4}}{5 \times V_{KMnO_4} \times \dfrac{M_{Na_2C_2O_4}}{1000}}$$

$$M_{Na_2C_2O_4} = 134.0$$

5. Notes

5.1　Commercial $KMnO_4$ can't be used directly to prepare a standard solution due to the existence of MnO_2 as an impurity, which can accelerate the decomposition of $KMnO_4$. MnO_2 must be eliminated by filtration, but filter paper cannot be used.

5.2　Distilled water generally contains some organic compounds, which can deoxidize $KMnO_4$, so the water must be boiled before use.

5.3　Light may accelerate the decomposition of $KMnO_4$, so a $KMnO_4$ solution must be preserved in a brown bottle and kept in dark place for 7～10 days.

5.4　The reaction is fairly slow, so the titration shouldn't be proceed too fast.

5.5　The temperature of the solution at the endpoint should not be less than 55 ℃.

6. Questions

1. Could HNO_3 and HCl be used to control acidity? Why?

2. What should be noticed when preparing a $KMnO_4$ solution？ Why?

实验十四　过氧化氢的含量测定

一、实验目的

1. 掌握用高锰酸钾标准溶液测定过氧化氢含量的原理和方法。
2. 掌握液体样品的取样方法。

二、实验原理

在酸性溶液中，高锰酸钾能氧化过氧化氢，过氧化氢发生还原反应，反应方程式如下：

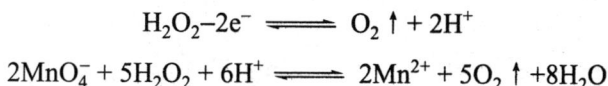

$$H_2O_2 - 2e^- \Longleftrightarrow O_2 \uparrow + 2H^+$$

$$2MnO_4^- + 5H_2O_2 + 6H^+ \Longleftrightarrow 2Mn^{2+} + 5O_2 \uparrow + 8H_2O$$

反应开始时速率很慢，而且溶液不容易褪色。当有少量二价锰离子生成时，反应速率则会加快。

三、仪器和材料

仪器　酸式滴定管（25 ml），锥形瓶（250 ml），移液管（1 ml），量筒（100 ml）。

材料　$KMnO_4$ 标准溶液（0.02 mol/L），硫酸溶液（1 mol/L），3%（W/V）过氧化氢溶液。

四、实验步骤

精密移取 1.00 ml 3%的过氧化氢溶液，置含有 20 ml 蒸馏水的 250 ml 锥形瓶中，再加入 20 ml 1 mol/L 的硫酸溶液，然后用 0.02 mol/L 高锰酸钾标准溶液滴定，直到终点显示浅红色。用滴定值计算过氧化氢含量：

$$H_2O_2(\%) = \frac{(CV)_{KMnO_4} \times 5 \times M_{H_2O_2}/1000}{2 \times V_{样品(ml)}} \times 100 (g/ml)$$

$$M_{H_2O_2} = 34.02$$

五、注意事项

过氧化氢受热易分解，因此滴定必须在室温下进行。

六、思考

1. 测定过氧化氢含量还有其他方法吗？

2. 当用高锰酸钾标准溶液测定过氧化氢溶液含量时，能采用硝酸、盐酸或醋酸控制酸度吗？为什么？

3. 采用高锰酸钾标准溶液测定过氧化氢的含量时，能否加热？为什么？

Experiment 14　Determination of Hydrogen Peroxide

1. Objective

1.1　Master the principle and operation of determination of hydrogen peroxide with $KMnO_4$ standard solution.

1.2　Master the sampling method of liquid sample.

2. Principle

In acidic solution, $KMnO_4$ can oxidize H_2O_2 and it can be reduced, and the reaction is:

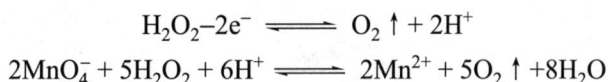

$$H_2O_2-2e^- \rightleftharpoons O_2\uparrow + 2H^+$$
$$2MnO_4^- + 5H_2O_2 + 6H^+ \rightleftharpoons 2Mn^{2+} + 5O_2\uparrow + 8H_2O$$

At the beginning of the reaction, the speed is slow, and the solution fades difficultly. When a small amount of Mn^{2+} is produced, the reaction speeds up by the auto catalytic of Mn^{2+}.

3. Apparatus and Materials

Apparatus: acid burette (25 ml), conical flask (250 ml), pipette (1 ml), cylinder (100 ml).

Materials: $KMnO_4$ standard solution (0.02 mol/L), H_2SO_4 solution (1 mol/L), 3%（W/V） H_2O_2 solution.

4. Procedures

Pipet out 1.00 ml of 3% (W/V) H_2O_2 solution into a 250 ml conical flask with 20 ml dislilled water. Add 20 ml of 1 mol/L H_2SO_4 solution, and titrate with 0.02 mol/L $KMnO_4$ standard solutions, until a faint but distinct reddish color is obtained.

From the titration value calculate the concentration of the H_2O_2 solution:

$$H_2O_2(\%)=\frac{(CV)_{KMnO_4}\times5\times M_{H_2O_2}/1000}{2\times V_{sample(ml)}}\times100(g/ml)$$

$$M_{H_2O_2} = 34.02$$

5. Notes

Because H_2O_2 readily decomposes when heated, the titration must be carried on under house temperature.

6. Questions

1. What other methods can be used to determine the concentration of H_2O_2?

2. When determine the concentration of H_2O_2 with $KMnO_4$ solution, Can HNO_3, HCl, and HAc be used to control acidity? Why?

3. Can the solution be heated when the content of H_2O_2 solution is measured with $KMnO_4$ standard solution? Why?

实验十五　硝酸银标准溶液的配制和标定

一、实验目的

1. 掌握莫尔法和佛尔哈德法的原理和方法。
2. 了解利用基准物质氯化钠标定硝酸银标准溶液的方法。
3. 学会正确判断铬酸钾指示剂终点。

二、实验原理

硝酸银溶液应用莫尔法进行标定，莫尔法是一种利用二次沉淀作为指示方法的直接标定方法。这种方法用纯氯化钠标定，铬酸钾为指示剂。

滴定开始前，向中性溶液中滴加少量铬酸钾，由于氯化银比铬酸银的溶解度小，所以氯化银先沉淀。接近滴定终点时，铬酸银生成并利用它的微红色判断终点。在铬酸银的红色显示之前，氯离子必须全部定量反应生成氯化银。滴定过程中发生的反应如下：

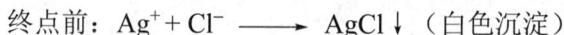

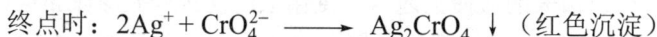

$$终点前：Ag^+ + Cl^- \longrightarrow AgCl\downarrow（白色沉淀）$$

$$终点时：2Ag^+ + CrO_4^{2-} \longrightarrow Ag_2CrO_4\downarrow（红色沉淀）$$

采用硝酸银滴定法，标定硫氰酸铵溶液时，铁铵矾作为指示剂。为了防止 Fe^{3+} 水解滴定应在酸性条件下进行。反应如下：

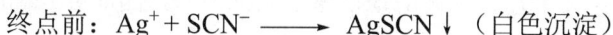

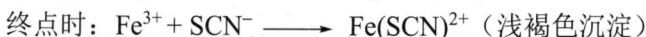

$$终点前：Ag^+ + SCN^- \longrightarrow AgSCN\downarrow（白色沉淀）$$

$$终点时：Fe^{3+} + SCN^- \longrightarrow Fe(SCN)^{2+}（浅褐色沉淀）$$

三、仪器和材料

仪器　酸式滴定管（25 ml），锥形瓶（250 ml），移液管（20 ml，1 ml），量筒（10 ml，100 ml），烧杯（250 ml），电子分析天平。

材料　硝酸银（A.R.），硫氰酸铵（A.R.），铬酸钾指示剂（5%水溶液），铁铵矾指示剂。

四、实验步骤

1. 0.1 mol/L 硝酸银溶液的配制　称取 17.5 g 硝酸银晶体，少量水溶解，然后稀释到大约 1000 ml，并在加塞棕色试剂瓶中振摇混合均匀。

2. 硝酸银溶液的标定　称取 0.1 g 的纯氯化钠，于 250 ml 的锥形瓶中并用 25 ml 水溶解。然后滴加 1 ml 5%铬酸钾溶液（建议用 1 ml 移液管）作为指示剂，然后置于白瓷砖上（避光），用 0.1 mol/L 的硝酸银滴定，不断振摇，直至产生红色。利用如下公式计算硝酸银的摩尔浓度。

$$C_{\mathrm{AgNO_3}} = \frac{W_{\mathrm{NaCl}}}{V_{\mathrm{AgNO_3}} \times \dfrac{M_{\mathrm{NaCl}}}{1000}}$$

$$M_{\mathrm{NaCl}} = 58.44$$

3. 0.1 mol/L 硫氰酸铵溶液的配制 称取 8 g 硫氰酸铵结晶，用少量水溶解稀释到 1000 ml，并置具塞玻璃瓶中混合至均匀。

4. 硫氰酸铵溶液的标定 精密移取 20.00 ml 硝酸银标准溶液，于 250 ml 锥形瓶中，加入 20 ml 蒸馏水、5 ml 6 mol/L 的硝酸和 2 ml 铁铵矾指示剂，然后用硫氰酸铵进行滴定，不断搅拌，直至在溶液出现红棕色。然后逐滴加入硫氰酸铵，并在每一滴加入后充分振摇，终点时显示持久的红色。再滴定两份，用以下式子计算硫氰酸铵的摩尔浓度：

$$C_{\mathrm{NH_4SCN}} = \frac{C_{\mathrm{AgNO_3}} \times V_{\mathrm{AgNO_3}}}{V_{\mathrm{NH_4SCN}}}$$

五、注意事项

1. 每步反应都应加入精确量的铬酸钾，以减少滴定误差。

2. 在滴定氯化钠的过程中，必须不断振摇，因为氯化银沉淀吸附的氯离子不能与银离子完全反应，否则，滴定终点可能明显提前。

3. 当铬酸银的红色消失的缓慢的时候，氯化银沉淀也开始凝聚，这说明大部分氯离子已形成沉淀，在这种情形下，硝酸银需要缓慢地逐滴加入并且充分振摇。

4. 滴定反应需要在中性或弱碱性溶液中进行，溶液 pH 最好控制在 7～10.5。

5. 水中不能含有氯离子，否则硝酸银溶液会是浑浊的，因而导致硝酸银溶液不能用。

六、思考

1. 利用不同的指示剂，有几种方法可以用来标定硝酸银溶液？指出每种方法的反应条件。

2. 铁铵矾指示剂如何配制？三氯化铁可以做指示剂吗？

Experiment 15　Preparation and Standardization of the Standard Silver Nitrate Solutions

1. Objective

1.1　Master the principles and the two methods of Mohr and Volhard.

1.2　Learn the method of standardization of the silver nitrate solution by the primary standard sodium chloride.

1.3　Judge correctly the end point of the potassium chromate indicator.

2. Principle

Silver nitrate ($AgNO_3$) solution is standardized with Mohr method, which is a direct titration method and uses a secondary precipitate as the indicator. The method is standardized by pure sodium chloride (NaCl), potassium chromate (K_2CrO_4) is used as an indicator.

At the beginning of the titration, a small amount of K_2CrO_4 is added to the neutral solution. AgCl being more insoluble than Ag_2CrO_4 firstly precipitated. At or near the equivalence point a precipitate of Ag_2CrO_4 is produced and this is recognized by its reddish color. The condition during the titration must be such the chloride is precipitated quantitatively as AgCl before the precipitation of the reddish silver chromate is perceptible. The reactions that take place during the titration may be expressed by the following equations:

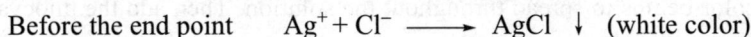

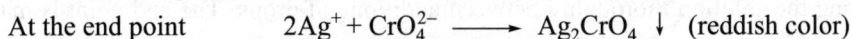

Before the end point　　$Ag^+ + Cl^- \longrightarrow AgCl \downarrow$　(white color)

At the end point　　$2Ag^+ + CrO_4^{2-} \longrightarrow Ag_2CrO_4 \downarrow$　(reddish color)

The ammonium thiocyanate (NH_4SCN) solution is standardized by the titration of $AgNO_3$ with ammonium ferric sulfate indicator. To prevent the hydrolysis of Fe^{3+}, the titration should be carried out in acid solution. The reaction is as follows:

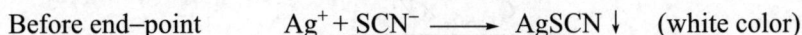

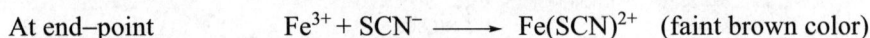

Before end–point　　$Ag^+ + SCN^- \longrightarrow AgSCN \downarrow$　(white color)

At end–point　　$Fe^{3+} + SCN^- \longrightarrow Fe(SCN)^{2+}$　(faint brown color)

3. Apparatus and Materials

Apparatus: acid burette (25 ml), conical flask (250 ml), pipette (20 ml, 1 ml), cylinder (10 ml, 100 ml), beaker (250 ml), electronic analytical balance.

Materials: $AgNO_3$ (A.R.), NH_4SCN (A.R.), K_2CrO_4 indicator solution (5% water solution), ammonium ferric sulfate indicator.

4. Procedures

4.1 Preparation of 0.1 mol/L AgNO₃ solution

Dissolve about 17.5 g (roughly weighed on the laboratory scales) of $AgNO_3$ crystals in a little water, dilute to about 1000 ml, and shake vigorously in a brown glass stoppered bottle to insure uniformity.

4.2 Standardization of AgNO₃ solution

Weigh out about 0.1 g pure NaCl into a 250 ml conical flasks, and dissolve in 25 ml of water. Add 1 ml of 5% K_2CrO_4 solution as indicator (preferably with 1 ml pipette), resting upon a white tile (away from sunlight), and slowly titrate with 0.1 mol/L $AgNO_3$ solution, swirling the liquid constantly, until a faint but distinct reddish color of the suspension is obtained. From the titration value calculate the molarity of the $AgNO_3$ solution:

$$C_{AgNO_3} = \frac{W_{NaCl}}{V_{AgNO_3} \times \frac{M_{NaCl}}{1000}}$$

$$M_{NaCl} = 58.44$$

4.3 Preparation of 0.1 mol/L NH₄SCN solution

Dissolve about 8 g (roughly weighed on the laboratory scales) of NH_4SCN crystals in a little water, dilute to about 1000 ml, and shake vigorously in a stoppered bottle to insure uniformity.

4.4 Standardization of NH₄SCN solution

Pipet 20.00 ml of standard $AgNO_3$ solution into a 250 ml conical flask. Add 20 ml of distilled water, 5 ml of 6 mol/L nitric acid, and 2 ml of iron (III) alum indicator solution (ammonium ferric sulfate indicator). Titrate with thiocyanate, swirling the solution constantly, until the reddish-brown color begins to spread throughout the solution. Then add the thiocyanate drop wise, shaking the solution thoroughly between additions of drops. The end point is marked by the permanent appearance of the reddish color of the iron-thiocyanate complex.

Titrate two additional portions of the silver nitrate solution with thiocyanate. Calculate the molarity of the thiocyanate solution.

$$C_{NH_4SCN} = \frac{C_{AgNO_3} \times V_{AgNO_3}}{V_{NH_4SCN}}$$

5. Notes

5.1 Every effort should be made to use exact amount of K_2CrO_4 indicator so as to reduce the titration error.

5.2 During the titration of NaCl, it is necessary to shake constantly because the chloride ions which are absorbed by precipitated AgCl do not react with silver ions completely. Otherwise, the end point may apparently be reached too early.

5.3　When the red color of silver chromate begins to disappear more slowly, and AgCl begins to agglomerate. It is indicated that most of NaCl has been precipitated. At this the $AgNO_3$ solution should be added slowly drop wise and shaken vigorously.

5.4　The titration must be carried out in neutral or weakly alkaline solution. The pH should begreater than 7, but not larger than 10.5.

5.5　The water should not contain Cl^-, otherwise the $AgNO_3$ solution would be turbid, and thus cannot be used.

6. Questions

1. How many methods can be used to standardize $AgNO_3$ solution with different indicators? Point out the conditions under which each of the methods is used.

2. How is iron (III) alum indicator prepared? Can $FeCl_3$ be used as indicator?

实验十六　氯化铵的含量测定

一、实验目的

1. 掌握吸附指示剂法的原理和操作方法。
2. 学会正确判断滴定终点。

二、实验原理

吸附指示剂法（法扬司法）是以吸附剂为指示剂的银量法。该法是利用沉淀对有机染料吸附而改变颜色来指示终点的方法。吸附指示剂是一类有色的有机染料，当它被带电的沉淀胶粒吸附时，因其结构改变而导致颜色改变，以此指示滴定终点。

氯化铵可用吸附指示剂法滴定，用 $AgNO_3$ 标准溶液为滴定液，荧光黄为指示剂。荧光黄（HFIn）在溶液中存在以下离解平衡：

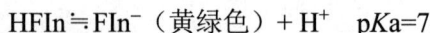

$$HFIn \rightleftharpoons FIn^- （黄绿色）+ H^+ \quad pKa=7$$

在化学计量点前，溶液中 Cl^- 过量，AgCl 表面吸附 Cl^-，不吸附 FIn^-。这一过程可用下式表示：$AgCl \cdot Cl^- + FIn^-$（黄绿色）。溶液呈 FIn^- 的黄绿色。

在化学计量点后，溶液中 Ag^+ 过量，AgCl 表面吸附 Ag^+ 带正电荷，带正电荷的胶团又吸附 FIn^-，被吸附后的 FIn^-，结构发生变化呈粉红色，从而指示终点。这一过程可用下式表示：$AgCl \cdot Ag^+ + FIn^- = AgCl \cdot Ag^+ \cdot FIn^-$（粉红色）。

三、仪器和材料

仪器　棕色酸式滴定管（25 ml），锥形瓶（250 ml），容量瓶（250 ml），移液管（25 ml），烧杯（50 ml），量筒（10 ml）。

材料　$AgNO_3$ 标准溶液（0.1 mol/L），NH_4Cl 样品，糊精溶液(1→50)，荧光黄指示剂。

四、实验步骤

准确称取氯化铵样品 1 g，加水溶解并配成 250 ml 溶液。准确吸取该溶液 25.00 ml 于 250 ml 锥形瓶中，加入 3 ml 2%(W/W)糊精溶液和 4～5 滴荧光黄指示剂，用 $AgNO_3$ 标准溶液（0.1 mol/L）滴定至颜色由黄绿色变为粉红色。滴定过程中要不断旋摇溶液并避免阳光和荧光灯直射。重复上述操作两次并按下式计算氯化铵含量。

$$NH_4Cl(\%) = \frac{(CV)_{AgNO_3} \times M_{NH_4Cl}/1000}{W_{NH_4Cl} \times \frac{25}{250}} \times 100\%$$

$$M_{NH_4Cl} = 53.49$$

五、注意事项

1. 在光的作用下，氯化银颜色会变暗，这是因为光可将氯化银轻微还原产生金属银并释放出氯气。银分散在氯化银胶体中使沉淀呈紫色。荧光灯也有明显的光化学效应。

2. 滴定过程中，由于氯离子被吸附在氯化银表面不易与银离子完全反应，所以必须不断振摇溶液，否则会提前到达终点。

3. 由于颜色变化发生在沉淀表面，沉淀的比表面积越大，终点变色越明显。因此，常加入保护胶体试剂如糊精等，使其保持胶体状态。

六、思考

1. 铬酸钾指示剂法或铁铵矾指示剂法能否用于氯化铵的含量测定，为什么？

2. 在氯化铵含量测定中为什么要加入糊精溶液？

Experiment 16　Determination of Ammonium Chloride

1. Objective

1.1　Master the principle and method of adsorption indicator method.

1.2　Learn how to judge the end point correctly.

2. Principle

The adsorption indicator method is a kind of argentimetry which is used adsorbent as indicator. This method is a method to indicate the end point by using precipitation to adsorb organic dyes and change colors. Adsorption indicator is a kind of colored organic dyes，when it is adsorbed by a charged precipitated colloid, the color changes due to the change in structure, thus indicating the titration end point.

Ammonium chloride can be titrated by adsorption indicator method, $AgNO_3$ is used as standard solution and fluorescence is used as an indicator. The fluorescence (HFIn) has the following dissociation equilibrium in the solution:

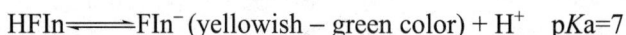

$$HFIn \Longrightarrow FIn^- (yellowish - green\ color) + H^+ \quad pKa=7$$

Before the stoichiometric point，chloride ions excess in solution. Silver chloride adsorbs Cl^- on its surface, but not adsorbs FIn^-，and the formula of the precipitate can be represented by the following: $AgCl \cdot Cl^- + FIn^-$(yellowish-green color). The solution assumes its normal yellowish-green color.

After the stoichiometric point，silver ions excess in solution. The surface of silver chloride adsorbs silver ions so that it has a positive charge on its surface. A positively charged micelle adsorbs fluoresceinate ions. After being adsorbed, the structure of the FIn^- is changed and the color turns reddish pink to indicate the end point. This procedure can be represented by the following formula: $AgCl \cdot Ag^+ + FIn^- \Longrightarrow AgCl \cdot Ag^+ \cdot FIn^-$ (reddish pink color).

3. Apparatus and Materials

Apparatus: brown acid burette (25 ml), conical flask (250 ml), volumetric flask (250 ml), pipette (25 ml), beaker (50 ml), cylinder (10 ml).

Materials: $AgNO_3$ standard solution(0.1 mol/L), NH_4Cl sample, dextrin solution (1→50), fluorescein indicator.

4. Procedures

Weigh out accurately about 1 g of ammonium chloride, dissolve in water and dilute to

250 ml. Pipet out 25.00 ml of the solution into a 250 ml conical flask, add 3 ml of 2%(W/W) dextrin solution and 4 or 5 drops of fluorescein indicator, and titrate the solution with AgNO₃ standard solution until the color changes from yellowish-green to pink. Swirl the solution during the titration, keep it away from direct sunlight and strong fluorescent light. Repeat the above operation twice and calculate the percentage of ammonium chloride as follows:

$$NH_4Cl(\%) = \frac{(CV)_{AgNO_3} \times M_{NH_4Cl}/1000}{W_{NH_4Cl} \times \dfrac{25}{250}} \times 100\%$$

$$M_{NH_4Cl} = 53.49$$

5. Notes

5.1　Under the action of light, the color of silver chloride darkens because light can slightly reduce silver chloride to metal silver and release chlorine. The precipitate then assumes a purplish color due to colloidal dispersion of the silver in the AgCl. Fluorescent light also has a marked photochemical effect.

5.2　During the titration of ammonium chloride, it is necessary to shake constantly because the chloride ions which are absorbed by precipitated silver chloride do not react with silver ions completely. Otherwise, the end point may apparently be reached too early.

5.3　Since the color change takes place on the surface of the particles, The larger the specific surface area of the precipitation, the more obvious the discoloration of the end point is. Therefore, protective colloidal reagents such as dextrin is often added to keep colloidal.

6. Questions

6.1　Can K_2CrO_4 indicator method or volhard method be used for the determination of ammonium chloride? Why?

6.2　Why is the dextrin solution added in the determination of ammonium chloride?

实验十七　自来水中氯含量的测定

一、实验目的

1. 了解沉淀滴定法测定水中微量氯离子含量的方法。
2. 学习沉淀滴定的基本操作。

二、实验原理

自来水中氯离子（Cl⁻）的定量检测，最常用的方法是莫尔法（沉淀滴定法）。该法是在中性或弱碱性介质（pH＝6.5～10.5）中，以 K_2CrO_4 为指示剂，用 $AgNO_3$ 标准溶液直接滴定 Cl⁻。由于 AgCl 的溶解度比 Ag_2CrO_4 的溶解度小，因此，在滴定过程中 AgCl 先沉淀出来。当 AgCl 定量沉淀后，微过量的 Ag^+ 与 CrO_4^{2-} 生成砖红色的 Ag_2CrO_4 沉淀，指示滴定终点。反应如下：

$$Ag^+ + Cl^- \rightleftharpoons AgCl\downarrow（白色）$$
$$2Ag^+ + CrO_4^{2-} \rightleftharpoons Ag_2CrO_4\downarrow（砖红色）$$

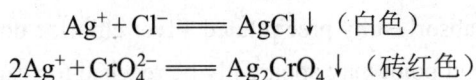

三、仪器与材料

仪器　酸式滴定管（棕色，10 ml），烧杯（100 ml，150 ml），移液管（10 ml），容量瓶（250 ml），锥形瓶（150 ml）。

材料　$AgNO_3$（A.R.），NaCl 基准试剂，K_2CrO_4 溶液（0.5%）。

四、实验步骤

1. $AgNO_3$ 标准溶液（0.005 mol/L）的配制与标定　称取 0.085 g $AgNO_3$ 溶解于 100 ml 不含 Cl⁻的蒸馏水中，摇匀，储存于带玻璃塞的棕色试剂瓶中于暗处保存，待标定。

准确称取 0.07～0.08 g NaCl 基准试剂于 100 ml 烧杯中，用适量蒸馏水溶解后，定量转移至 250 ml 容量瓶中，定容。准确移取此溶液 10.00 ml 于 150 ml 锥形瓶中，加入 1 滴 K_2CrO_4（0.5%）溶液，不断振摇下，用 $AgNO_3$ 溶液进行滴定至溶液呈砖红色即为终点。记下消耗的 $AgNO_3$ 溶液的体积，平行测定三次，计算 $AgNO_3$ 溶液的准确浓度。

2. 自来水中 Cl⁻离子的含量测定　准确量取 10.00 ml 水样于 150 ml 锥形瓶中，加入 1～2 滴 K_2CrO_4 溶液（0.5%），不断振摇下，用 $AgNO_3$ 溶液进行滴定至溶液呈砖红色即为终点。记下消耗的 $AgNO_3$ 溶液的体积，平行测定三次，计算自来水中 Cl⁻离子的含量（g/L）。

五、注意事项

1. 用 $AgNO_3$ 溶液进行滴定时应剧烈振摇，使 AgCl 沉淀吸附的 Cl⁻能够及时释放，防止滴定终点提前。

2. 实验结束后，含银废液应进行回收处理，不能倒入水槽中。

六、思考

1. 使用莫尔法时，K_2CrO_4 指示剂的用量过多或过少，对测定结果有何影响？
2. 使用莫尔法时，能否用标准 NaCl 溶液直接滴定 Ag^+ 离子？

Experiment 17　The Determination of the Content of Chlorine in Tap Water

1. Objective

1.1　Learn to determine the content of chlorine in tap water using precipitation titration.

1.2　Master the principle and method of precipitation titration.

2. Principle

The most commonly used method for the quantitative determination of chloride (Cl^-) in tap water is the Mohr method (precipitation titration). In neutral or alkalescent condition (pH = $6.5 \sim 10.5$), Cl^- in the test solution is direct titrated by $AgNO_3$ standard solution with K_2CrO_4 as indicator. Since the solubility of AgCl is smaller than that of Ag_2CrO_4, AgCl first precipitates during titration. When AgCl precipitated quantitatively, excessive Ag^+ reacts with CrO_4^{2-} to form a brick-red precipitation Ag_2CrO_4, indicating the endpoint of the titration. The titration reactions are as follows:

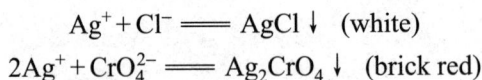

$$Ag^+ + Cl^- \Longrightarrow AgCl \downarrow \ \text{(white)}$$
$$2Ag^+ + CrO_4^{2-} \Longrightarrow Ag_2CrO_4 \downarrow \ \text{(brick red)}$$

3. Apparatus and Materials

Apparatus: acid burette (10 ml), beakers (100 ml, 150 ml), pipette (10 ml), volumetric flask (250 ml), erlenmeyer flask (150 ml).

Materials: $AgNO_3$ (A.R.), NaCl reference reagent, K_2CrO_4 solution (0.5%).

4. Procedures

4.1　Preparation and standardization of $AgNO_3$ standard solution (0.005 mol/L)

Weigh 0.085 g of $AgNO_3$ to a 150 ml beaker, add 100 ml of distilled water without Cl^- and mix well. Transfer the $AgNO_3$ solution to a brown reagent bottle with glass stopper and store in the dark.

Weigh accurately $0.07 \sim 0.08$ g of NaCl reference reagent to a 100 ml breaker, add appropriate amount of distilled water without Cl^- and transfer to a 250 ml volumetric flask, and mix well. Pipette accurately 10.00 ml of NaCl solution to an 150 ml erlenmeyer flask, add 1 drop of K_2CrO_4 solution (0.5%), and mix well. Under constant shaking, titrate the NaCl solution with $AgNO_3$ standard solution until the color of the solution is brick red. Repeat the procedure three times. Record the volume of the consumed AgNO$_3$ standard solution and calculate its concentration.

4.2　Determination of chlorine in tap water

Measure accurately 10.00 ml tap water to an 150 ml erlenmeyer flask, add 1～2 drops of K$_2$CrO$_4$ solution (0.5%), and mix well. Under constant shaking, titrate the tap water with AgNO$_3$ standard solution until the color of the solution is brick red. Repeat the procedure three times. Record the volume of the consumed AgNO$_3$ standard solution and calculate the content (g/L) of chlorine in tap water.

5. Notes

5.1　The titration with AgNO$_3$ solution should be under constant shaking vigorously to avoid the advancement of the endpoint.

5.2　Silver-containing wastewater should be recycled.

6. Questions

6.1　What is the effect if the amount of K$_2$CrO$_4$ indicator is too much or too little by Mohr method?

6.2　Whether Ag$^+$ can be direct titrated using NaCl standard solution by Mohr method?

实验十八　氯化钡中结晶水测定

一、实验目的

1. 熟悉重量分析的基本操作。
2. 了解结晶化合物结晶水的测量方法。

二、实验原理

烘箱干燥是测定固体含水量最简便的方法。结晶水合物（如 $BaCl_2 \cdot 2H_2O$）中的水分可采用重量分析法测定。当已知重量的样品在适当的温度下加热时（干燥直至样品重量恒定），其含水量应为加热前后其重量的差异。

$BaCl_2 \cdot 2H_2O$ 可在 113 ℃时失去结晶水，此温度下，$BaCl_2$ 非常稳定，不挥发或分解。因此，本实验温度高于 113 ℃。

$BaCl_2 \cdot 2H_2O$ 理论结晶水含量为 $14.75\% \left(\dfrac{2 \times 18.02}{244.27} \right)$，测得值应在 $14.75\% \pm 0.05\%$ 范围内。

$BaCl_2 \cdot 2H_2O$ 结晶水含量计算式：结晶水$\% = \dfrac{\text{干燥失重}(g)}{\text{样品重}(g)} \times 100\%$

三、仪器和材料

仪器　分析天平，称量瓶（扁平型），电热干燥箱，干燥器。

材料　$BaCl_2 \cdot 2H_2O$（A.R.）。

四、实验步骤

1. 称量瓶恒重　取 3 个洁净的称量瓶置于 115 ℃烘箱中烘干至少 1 h。之后把称量瓶放在干燥器中（在热的情况下，称量瓶盖不要盖严，以免冷却后不易打开），冷却至室温（30 min），取出并准确称其重量。重复以上操作直至恒重（两次质量之差≤0.3 mg）。

2. 烘去结晶水　分别称取约 1 g 的 $BaCl_2 \cdot 2H_2O$ 于已恒重的称量瓶中，并称重。将盛有试样的称量瓶置于 115 ℃的烘箱中，保持 1 h 后，将称量瓶转移至干燥器中，冷却至室温（30 min）后，称定其重量；然后进行第二次烘干（30 min），直至恒重。由烘干前后称量瓶和试样质量的差，即得出 $BaCl_2 \cdot 2H_2O$ 中结晶水的质量。

五、注意事项

1. 在样品恒重过程中，应注意平行原则，即称量瓶（或加样品后）加热干燥的温度及在干燥器中冷却的时间应保持一致。

2. 称量应迅速，以免干燥样品久置空气中吸潮而影响恒重。

六、思考

1. 空称量瓶为何要干燥至恒重？
2. 做好本实验有哪几个关键步骤？

Experiment 18   Determination of Water in Barium Chloride Dihydrate

1. Objective

1.1   Learn the basic operation of gravimetric analysis.

1.2   Know the measurement method of water in crystalline compounds.

2. Principle

Drying oven is the most convenient method for determining the water content of a solid. The water in a crystalline hydrate such as $BaCl_2 \cdot 2H_2O$ is readily determined gravimetrically. When a known weight sample is heated at a suitable temperature, its water content is taken as the difference in its weight before and after heating. The drying process is continued until the weight of the sample becomes constant at the chosen temperature.

The water of crystallization in $BaCl_2 \cdot 2H_2O$ will be lost at 113 ℃. At this temperature $BaCl_2$ is very stable because it is not volatilized or decomposed. So temperature higher than 113 ℃ can be applied in this experiment.

The theoretical percentage of crystallization water %=14.75%(2×18.02/244.24)

The practical percentage of crystallization water % = weight lost(g)/sample weight(g)×100%

3. Apparatus and Materials

Apparatus: analytical balance, weighing bottles, drying oven, desiccator.

Materials: $BaCl_2 \cdot 2H_2O$ (A.R.).

4. Procedures

4.1   Drying the weighing bottles to constant weight

Carefully clean two or three weighing bottles. Dry them for at least 1 h at 115 ℃ in drying oven. Weigh each bottle after it has cooled to room temperature (30 min) in desiccator. Repeat this cycle of heating, cooling, and weighing until the change of two successive weights is within the range of 0.3 mg.

4.2   Weighing of crystalline substances

Next, the approximate amount of each sample of $BaCl_2 \cdot 2H_2O$ (1 g) should be introduced to individual weighing bottles and reweighed. Heat the bottles with samples for about 1 h at 115 ℃; then cool in the desiccator for at least 30 min, and weigh the bottles as before. Repeat the heating cycle until constant weights for the bottles and their contents have been attained. Report the percentage of water in the sample, according to the difference in its weight before and after heating.

5. Notes

5.1　In the course of weighing a sample to constant weight, pay attention to the parallel principle such as the same cool time in desiccator, the same temperature in drying oven, and so on.

5.2　Weigh sample quickly to avoid absorbing water during weighing.

6. Questions

6.1　Why must the empty bottle be dried to constant weight?

6.2　What are the key steps in this experiment?

实验十九　磷酸的电位滴定

一、实验目的

1. 掌握电位滴定操作及确定化学计量点的方法。
2. 学会采用电位滴定法测定弱酸 pKa 的方法。

二、实验原理

电位滴定法的装置和操作都较一般容量滴定法繁琐，但对某些一般容量滴定不能进行的测定，如被测溶液混浊，溶液本身有颜色等，可用电位滴定法测定。此外，电位滴定法也可用来测定某些弱酸（或弱碱）的离解常数。

1. 离解常数 pK_a 的测定　磷酸为多元酸，其 pK_a 可用电位滴定法求得。离解常数 K_a 值即是半中和点时溶液中氢离子浓度。当 H_3PO_4 的第一个 H^+ 被滴定一半时，$[H_3PO_4]$ = $[H_2PO_4^-]$，则 K_{a_1} = $[H^+]$，即 pK_{a_1} = pH。同理，当第二个 H^+ 被中和一半时，$[H_2PO_4^-]$ = $[HPO_4^{2-}]$，则 K_{a_2} = $[H^+]$，即 pK_{a_2} = pH。

绘制 pH–V 滴定曲线，确定化学计量点。化学计量点一半的体积（半中和点的体积）对应的 pH 值，即为 H_3PO_4 的 pK_a。

2. 滴定终点的确定　电位滴定法确定滴定终点有多种方法。其中最直接的方法是绘制 pH–V 曲线，曲线的转折点即为终点。导数法在确定终点时可以提高准确度。一阶导数是计算滴定剂单位体积变化引起 pH 单位的变化值，即 $\Delta pH/\Delta V$；该曲线是以滴定剂体积的平均值为横坐标，一阶导数为纵坐标，其曲线的最高点即为终点。

三、仪器和材料

仪器　精密 pH 计，复合电极，电磁搅拌器，聚四氟乙烯搅拌棒，滴定管（25 ml），烧杯（100 ml），移液管（10 ml）。

材料　NaOH 标准溶液（0.1 mol/L），磷酸溶液（0.1 mol/L），混合磷酸盐标准缓冲溶液（pH 6.86），邻苯二甲酸氢钾标准缓冲溶液（0.05 mol/L，pH 4.00）。

四、实验步骤

1. pH 计的校准　用 0.05 mol/L 邻苯二甲酸氢钾标准缓冲溶液（pH 4.00）校准 pH 计。

2. 磷酸的滴定　精密量取磷酸样品溶液 15 ml，置 100 ml 烧杯中，加蒸馏水 10 ml，插入电极和搅拌子。测定磷酸溶液的 pH 值；开启电磁搅拌器；用 0.1 mol/L NaOH 液滴定，每加 2 ml 记录 pH 值，在接近化学计量点时，每加入一滴（如 0.1 ml 或 0.05 ml），记录一次 pH 值，继续滴定直至过了第二个化学计量点时为止。

3. 数据处理

（1）按 pH–V，$\Delta\text{pH}/\Delta V$–$\bar{V}$ 及 $\Delta^2\text{pH}/\Delta V^2$–$V$ 法作图，确定化学计量点，并计算 H_3PO_4 的浓度。

（2）根据 pH–V 曲线确定出 H_3PO_4 的 pK_{a_1} 和 pK_{a_2}；计算 H_3PO_4 的 K_{a_1} 和 K_{a_2}。

五、注意事项

1. 滴定剂加入后，要充分搅拌溶液以使溶液达到平衡。

2. 搅拌速率适当，避免滴定液的溅出。

3. 滴定过程中尽量少用蒸馏水冲洗，防止溶液过度稀释突跃不明显。

六、思考

1. 为什么磷酸的滴定曲线上只有两个滴定突跃？

2. 用 NaOH 滴定 H_3PO_4，第一化学计量点和第二化学计量点所消耗的 NaOH 体积理应相等，为什么实际上并不相等？

3. 滴定速率对实验结果是否有影响？

Experiment 19　The Potentiometric Titration of Phosphoric Acid

1. Objective

1.1　Master the operation of the potentiometric titration and the method of the judgement of the stoichiometric point.

1.2　Learn the method of determination of pK_a of the weak acid by potentiometric titration.

2. Principle

All the installation and operation of potentiometric titration are more trouble than a general capacity titration, but it has unique advantages with the turbid or colored solution. In addition, the dissociation constant of weak acid (or weak base) can be determined by potentiometric titration.

2.1　Determination of dissociation constants (pK_a)

Phosphoric acid is polyprotic acid whose pK_a can be obtained by potentiometric titration. A numerical value of K_a is derived from the pH at the point of half–neutralization. In the titration of H_3PO_4, we may assume that at the first midpoint, $[H_3PO_4] = [H_2PO_4^-]$ and $K_{a_1} = [H_3O^+]$ or $pK_{a_1} = pH$. When the second hydrogen of phosphoric acid is half–neutralization, $[H_2PO_4^-] = [HPO_4^{2-}]$, and $K_{a_2} = [H_3O^+]$ or $pK_{a_2} = pH$.

Draw the pH–V titration curve to determine the stoichiometric point. The pH value corresponding to the volume of the half of the stoichiometric point is the pK_a of H_3PO_4.

2.2　Determination of end point

The end point of a potentiometric titration can be determined by several methods. A direct method is the curve of pH versus titrant volume and the end point is given by finding the point of steep slope. A derivative method may improve the accuracy in locating the end point. First derivative is to calculate the change in pH per unit change in volume of titrant ($\Delta pH/\Delta V$). A plot of this parameter as a function of average volume leads to a sharp maximum at the end point.

3. Apparatus and Materials

Apparatus: pH meter, compound electrode, electromagnetic stirrer, a Teflon–coated stirring bar, burette (25 ml), beaker (100 ml), pipet (10 ml).

Materials: NaOH standard solution (0.1 mol/L), phosphoric acid solution (0.1 mol/L), mixed phosphate standard buffer solution (pH 6.86), potassium hydrogen phthalate standard buffer solution (0.05 mol/L, pH 4.00).

4. Procedures

4.1 Calibrate the pH meter

Calibrate the pH meter with 0.05 mol/L of potassium hydrogen phthalate standard buffer solution, pH 4.00.

4.2 Titration of phosphoric acid

Into a 100 ml beaker, pipet 15.00 m! of 0.1 mol/L phosphoric acid solution and dilute with 10 ml of distilled water. Place the electrode and a magnetic stirring bar into the beaker. Determine the pH value of the phosphoric acid solution (0.1 mol/L). Switch on magnetic stirrer, add NaOH solution from burette and record the readings of pH after each addition. At the outset, add large volumes (2 ml at a time), but reduce the additions to 0.10 ml or 0.05 ml in the vicinity of stoichiometric points. Titration is over after the second stoichiometric point.

4.3 Data processing

4.3.1 Draw the graph according to pH$-V$, ΔpH/$\Delta V-\overline{V}$, Δ^2pH/ΔV^2-V, determine the stoichiometric point, and calculate the concentration of H_3PO_4.

4.3.2 Determine pK_{a_1} and pK_{a_2} of H_3PO_4 according to the pH$-V$ curve, and calculate the K_{a_1} and K_{a_2} of H_3PO_4.

5. Notes

5.1 After each addition of titrant, sufficient time must be required for reaching equilibrium.

5.2 Choose a proper speed of stirring to avoid the splash of titrate.

5.3 The end point is sharper for more concentrated solutions. Consequently, avoid using more water to wash electrodes.

6. Questions

1. Why do only two titration jumps obtain from the titration curve of H_3PO_4 ?

2. Using NaOH titrate H_3PO_4, the consumed volume of NaOH between the first stoichiometric point and the second stoichiometric point should be the same size, however, the consumed volume are not equal actually, why?

3. Does titration rate have any effect on the experimental results?

实验二十　用氟离子选择电极测定水中氟离子含量

一、实验目的

1. 掌握电位法的基本原理。
2. 掌握离子选择性电极测量方法及数据处理方法。
3. 掌握离子计的使用方法。

二、实验原理

氟离子选择性电极（简称氟电极）是晶体膜电极，其电极膜由 LaF_3 单晶制成，内装有 NaF–NaCl 内参比溶液，以 Ag–AgCl 作内参比电极。将氟离子选择性电极（指示电极）和饱和甘汞电极（参比电极）插入到含氟的待测溶液中构成化学电池，测得的电动势随着溶液氟浓度的变化而变化，电池的电动势可用下式表示：$E = K - \dfrac{2.303RT}{F} \times \lg \alpha_{F^-}$，若在溶液中加入离子强度调节剂（TISAB），则氟离子的活度可用浓度代替，在 25 ℃时上式可写成：$E = K' - 0.059 \times \lg C_{F^-}$，当溶液 pH 范围在 5～7 之间，氟的浓度在 10^{-6}～10^{-1} mol/L 之间时，电动势和 $\lg C_{F^-}$ 呈良好的线性关系。所以本实验可采用工作曲线法和标准加入法测定水溶液中 F⁻ 含量。

三、仪器和材料

仪器　酸度计，电磁搅拌器，氟离子选择性电极（使用前应在 10^{-4} mol/L 的 F⁻溶液中浸泡活化 1～2 h），饱和甘汞电极。

材料　NaF 标准溶液（0.1 mol/L），TISAB 溶液（58 g NaCl，12 g 柠檬酸钠溶于去离子水中，加 57.0 ml 冰醋酸和 500 ml 去离子水，用 6 mol/L NaOH 调节 pH 至 5.0～5.5，加去离子水稀释至 1000 ml），自来水样。

四、实验步骤

1. 清洗电极　安装好氟电极和饱和甘汞电极，开启仪器开关，预热仪器，调好酸度计的 mV 档，将两电极浸入去离子水中，用蒸馏水清洗数次使测得的氟电极的电极电位至空白值 350 mV 以上。

2. 系列浓度标准溶液的配制　用移液管移取 5.00 ml 0.1 mol/L NaF 标准溶液于 50 ml 容量瓶，加入 5.00 ml TISAB 溶液，用蒸馏水定容至刻度，摇匀，得 10^{-2} mol/L NaF 标准溶液，采用逐级稀释法依次配制出浓度为 10^{-3} mol/L、10^{-4} mol/L、10^{-5} mol/L、10^{-6} mol/L 的 NaF 标准溶液各 50 ml，每次加 TISAB 溶液 4.5 ml 即可。

3. 工作曲线的测绘　将配制好的标准溶液分别倒入干燥的小烧杯中，按由稀到浓的顺序在搅拌下依次测量出各个溶液对应的电位值，每次测定不需清洗电极，只需用滤纸吸干即可。然后以测得的电动势 E（mV）为纵坐标，以$-\lg C_F$为横坐标，在坐标纸上绘制出工作曲线。

4. 样品中氟离子含量的测定　将电极用蒸馏水洗至空白电位值，把 5.00 ml TISAB 加入到 50 ml 容量瓶中，用样品定容至刻度，把样品溶液一次全部转入干净干燥的烧杯内，测定电动势，然后加入 0.50 ml 10^{-2} mol/L 的 NaF 标准溶液后再测一次电动势。分别用工作曲线法和标准加入法求算样品溶液中氟离子的含量。

五、注意事项

1. 测量时必须确保标准溶液由低到高依次进行，且每次更换溶液时用被测溶液清洗烧杯。
2. 测定样品前应用蒸馏水洗电极电位至空白值，避免产生较大误差。
3. 测定过程时搅拌速度应该缓慢而稳定。
4. 不得用手触摸电极的敏感膜。

六、思考

1. 本实验中加入离子强度调节剂的目的是什么？
2. 绘制工作曲线时，为什么氟标准溶液按由低到高的顺序测量？
3. 为什么清洗氟电极，使其相应电位值大于 350 mV 以上？

Experiment 20　Determination of F⁻ in Water by Fluorine Ion-Selective Electrode

1. Objective

1.1　Master the basic principle of potential method.
1.2　Master the measuring method and data processing method of ion-selective electrode.
1.3　Maste the operation of the ion-meter.

2. Principle

The fluorine ion selective electrode is crystal membrane electrode. Electrode membrane is composed of a crystal LaF_3 thin membrane. The internal reference is Ag–AgCl electrode filled with NaF–NaCl solution. External reference electrode is saturated calomel electrode. Both the fluorine ion-selective electrode and the reference electrode are inserted into analyte solution containing fluoride. If the concentration of F⁻ in the analyte solution changes, the voltage measured between the two reference electrodes also changes. The electromotive force of the battery is represented by the following formula.

$$E = K - \frac{2.303RT}{F} \times \lg \alpha_{F^-}$$

If TISAB solution is added into the solution, the activity of fluorine ion can be replaced by the concentration of fluorine ion. So at 25 ℃ the above formula can be written again as follows:

$$E = K' - 0.059 \times \lg C_{F^-}$$

At pH5～7, when the concentration of fluorine is between 10^{-6}～10^{-1} mol/L, there is a good linear relationship between the electrode potential and the concentration. Therefore, the work curve method and standard addition method can be used to determine the content of F⁻ the aqueous solution.

3. Apparatus and Materials

Apparatus: acidity–meter, electromagnetic stirrer, fluorine ion–selective electrode (It should be soaked in 10^{-4} mol/L F⁻ solution for 1～2 hours before use), saturated calomel electrode (SCE).

Materials: NaF stock standard solution (0.1000 mol/L), TISAB solution (weigh 58 g of sodium chloride, 12 g of sodium citrate, dissolved in deionized water, add 57.0 ml of glacial acetic acid and 500 ml of deionized water, adjust pH to 5.0～5.5 with 6 mol/L NaOH, then dilute to 1000 ml with deionized water), tap water sample.

4. Procedures

4.1 Cleaning electrode

Install the fluorine ion–selective electrode and saturated calomel electrode. Open the equipment switch, preheating instrument. Adjust pH meter to mV file. Wash fluoride electrode with distilled water several times to make the electrode potential of the fluorine electrode above 350 mV.

4.2 Preparation of a series of the NaF standard solutions

Pipet 5.00 ml of 0.1000 mol/L NaF standard solution to a 50 ml volumetric flask, add 5.00 ml TISAB solution, dilute to the mark with distilled water, mix well. The standard solution of 10^{-2} mol/L NaF is obtained. The standard NaF solution of 10^{-3} mol/L, 10^{-4} mol/L, 10^{-5} mol/L, 10^{-6} mol/L can be prepared by step by step dilution method and 50 ml of each NaF standard solution is obtained. 4.5 ml TISAB solution can be added at a time.

4.3 Mapping working curve

According to the concentration of the series of the NaF standard solutions, from thin to thick, transfer each solution into the dry beaker. The corresponding potential values of each solution are measured in turn under stirring. Each time the electrode is not washed, only filter paper is used to dry it. Then the measured electromotive force E(mV) is taken as the ordinate. Take $\lg C_{F^-}$ as the abscissa, the working curve is drawn on the coordinate paper.

4.4 Determination of the content of fluoride ion in aqueous sample

Wash the electrode potential to a blank value using distilled water. Add 5.00 ml of TISAB solution to a 50 ml volumetric flask, dilute with sample to scale. Pour this sample into a dry beaker, and determine its electromotive force value. Add 0.50 ml NaF standard solutions (1.00×10^{-2} mol/L) to the beaker, mix well. Determine its electromotive force value again under stirring.

Working curve method and the standard addition method are respectively used to calculate fluorine ion content of sample solution.

5. Notes

5.1   The measurement order should be from low to high, and the beaker should be cleaned while the solution is replaced.

5.2   In order to avoid large error, the electrode potential should be washed to a blank value with distilled water before determination.

5.3   The speed of stirring should be slow and steady during the measuring process.

5.4   Do not touch the electrode film by hand.

6. Questions

1. What is the purpose of adding TISAB solution in this experiment?

2. Why is the standard solution measured in order from low to high when drawing the working curve?

3. Why can the fluorine electrode be cleaned so that the corresponding potential is greater than 350 mV?

实验二十一 永停滴定法标定 I_2 标准溶液

一、实验目的

1. 掌握永停滴定法的原理及其操作。
2. 掌握永停滴定终点的判断方法。
3. 熟悉永停滴定法的装置。

二、实验原理

永停滴定法属于电流滴定法，是将两支相同的铂电极插入到待测溶液中，外加一个小电压（10～200 mV），在滴定过程中通过观察两电极之间电流的变化来确定滴定终点，永停滴定法仪器装置简单，操作方便，结果准确可靠。

本实验用硫代硫酸钠标准溶液滴定 I_2 溶液，用永停滴定法确定滴定终点，滴定反应式如下：$I_2 + 2S_2O_3^{2-} \rightleftharpoons 2I^- + S_4O_6^{2-}$，在化学计量点之前，溶液里有 I_2/I^- 可逆电对，存在电流。随着滴定的进行，I_2 的浓度逐渐变小，电流也逐渐减小。当化学计量点时，电流降到最低；化学计量点后，加入稍过量的硫代硫酸钠，溶液里只有不可逆电对 $S_4O_6^{2-}/S_2O_3^{2-}$ 存在，电流计指针停留在 0。这种类型的滴定是以电流计指针突然下降至 0 并不再改变来确定滴定终点，根据消耗的 $Na_2S_2O_3$ 的体积，计算出 I_2 的浓度。

三、仪器和材料

仪器 自动永停滴定仪（ZTX-1），Pt 电极，酸式滴定管（25 ml），烧杯（100 ml），移液管（5 ml），铁心搅拌棒。

材料 I_2 标准溶液（0.005 mol/L），$Na_2S_2O_3$ 标准溶液（0.01 mol/L），KI（A.R.）。

四、实验步骤

1. 根据说明书连接仪器，调节极化电压在 10～15 mV。
2. 准确移取 5 ml 碘溶液放入 100 ml 烧杯中，加 0.1 g KI，稀释至 50 ml。用 0.01 mol/L $Na_2S_2O_3$ 标准溶液边搅拌边滴定，每滴定 0.5 ml 记录电流值，当碘溶液变成浅黄色时（接近化学计量点时），每滴定 0.2 ml 或 0.1 ml 记录电流值，直至电流保持不变。
3. 绘制 I—V 曲线，通过曲线记录在化学计量点消耗的 $Na_2S_2O_3$ 的体积，计算碘溶液浓度。

五、注意事项

1. 实验前，检查永停滴定仪线路连接和外加电压。
2. 使用前应该活化铂电极，在含有少量 $FeCl_3$ 的浓硝酸溶液中至少浸泡半小时，浸泡时勿接触器皿底部，以免弯折受损。

3. 实验结束时，要把检流计和永停装置电流切断，以免损坏仪器。

六、思考

1. 永停滴定法和电位滴定在原理上有何不同？

2. 在滴定过程中如果加的电压过高会发生什么现象？

3. 外指示剂和永停滴定法两者确定终点方法的优缺点有哪些？

Experiment 21　Standardization of I₂ Standard Solution by Dead-stop Titration Method

1. Objective

1.1　Master the principle and operation of dead-stop titration.

1.2　Master the determination of the end point of dead-stop titration.

1.3　Familiar with the instrument of dead-stop titration.

2. Principle

Dead-stop titration belongs to amperometric titration. Insert two identical Pt electrodes into the test solution and apply a low voltage ($10\sim200$ mV) between the two electrodes, then the titration end point can be determined through observing the change of current during the titration process. This method has the virtue of simple apparatus, easy operation and accurate result.

In this experiment, the $Na_2S_2O_3$ standard solution is used for titrating I_2 solution, and the titration end point is determined by dead-stop titration method. The titration reaction is as follow:

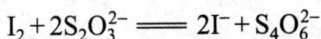

$$I_2 + 2S_2O_3^{2-} = 2I^- + S_4O_6^{2-}$$

Before stoichiometric point, the reversible electric couples, I_2/I^-, is present in the test solution, so an electrolysis current flows through the two electrodes. With the proceeding of titration, the concentration of I_2 becomes lower, and the current also becomes smaller. At stoichiometric point, the current reduces to minimum. After stoichiometric point, only the nonreversible electric couples, $S_4O_6^{2-}/S_2O_3^{2-}$, and I^- are present in the solution, there is no electrolytic reaction, and also no change in current. Hence, the titration end point is determined by dropping to zero and holding no change of the galvanometer needle. According to the volume of $Na_2S_2O_3$, the concentration of I_2 is calculated.

3. Apparatus and Materials

Apparatus: automatic dead–stop titration instrument (ZTX–1), Pt electrodes, burette (25 ml), beaker (100 ml), pipet (5 ml), magnetic stirrer.

Materials: I_2 solution (0.005 mol/L), $Na_2S_2O_3$ standard solution (0.01 mol/L), KI (A.R.).

4. Procedures

4.1　Connect wires correctly according to the instruction, and adjust the voltage at the region $10\sim15$ mV.

4.2   Transfer accurately 5 ml of I_2 solution into a 100 ml beaker, add 0.1 g of KI and dilute to 50 ml with distilled water. Titrate with 0.01 mol/L of $Na_2S_2O_3$ standard solution under stirring, and record current value I every addition of 0.5 ml. When the solution of I_2 shows pale-yellow, it indicates the stoichiometric point will approach, thus be careful with titration. Record current value I every addition 0.2 ml or 0.1 ml until the reading remains unchanged.

4.3   Draw the I—V curve, record the volume of $Na_2S_2O_3$ consumed at the stoichiometric point on the curve, and then calculate the concentration of I_2 solution.

5. Notes

5.1   Before the experiment, check the voltage applied on the galvanometer and the junction of the circuitry.

5.2   Before use, Pt electrodes are activated. Soak them in concentrated nitric acid containing a small amount of $FeCl_3$ at least 30 min, and do not touch the bottom of beaker in order to avoid being bent.

5.3   Turn off the power of the galvanometer and the dead-stop apparatus so as not to damage the instrument.

6. Questions

1. What are the differences in principle between dead–stop titration and potentiometric titration?

2. What happens if the voltage is too high during titration?

3. What are the advantages and disadvantages of the indicator method and the dead-stop method for determining the end point?

实验二十二　紫外-可见分光光度法测定维生素 B_{12} 注射液的含量

一、实验目的

1. 掌握绘制吸收曲线的方法及选择波长的原则。
2. 掌握紫外-可见分光光度仪的使用方法和注意事项。
3. 掌握吸收系数法测定组分含量的方法。

二、实验原理

吸收曲线又叫吸收光谱，是以波长 λ（nm）为横坐标，以吸光度 A（或透光率 T）为纵坐标绘制的曲线。当建立紫外-可见分光光度法用于含量测定时，首先应绘制该物质的吸收曲线。通常应选被测物质吸收光谱中的吸收峰处的波长，以提高灵敏度并减小测量误差。如果被测物质有几个吸收峰，可选无其他物质干扰的、较高的吸收峰。一般不选择光谱中靠短波长末端的吸收峰。本实验采用连续变换分光光度计的测定波长来绘制维生素 B_{12} 的吸收曲线。

单组分样品的含量测定方法有吸收系数法、工作曲线法和对照法。本实验采用的是吸收系数法测定维生素 B_{12} 注射液的含量。维生素 B_{12} 分子结构中含有钴元素，因此它的注射液为粉红色至红色的澄明液体。维生素 B_{12} 有三个吸收峰，分别位于在 278 nm、361 nm 和 550 nm。其中 361 nm 吸收峰最高，并且干扰较少。因此，361 nm 波长处的吸收系数（ $E_{1cm}^{1\%} = 207$ ）可用作计算其含量。

三、仪器和材料

仪器　紫外-可见分光光度计，容量瓶（10 ml），移液管（1 ml）。
材料　维生素 B_{12} 水溶液（0.1 mg/ml）；维生素 B_{12} 注射液。

四、实验步骤

1. 维生素 B_{12} 吸收曲线的绘制　取适量 0.1 mg/ml 维生素 B_{12} 溶液于 1 cm 比色皿中，以蒸馏水为空白溶液，测定 340～580 nm 范围内的吸光度。其中 340～370 nm 和 540～580 nm 每 5 nm 间隔测量一次，其余每 20 nm 间隔测量一次。以测定波长为横坐标，吸光度为纵坐标绘制维生素 B_{12} 的吸收曲线。

2. 维生素 B_{12} 注射液的含量测定　精密量取维生素 B_{12} 注射液适量，加水定量稀释成维生素 B_{12} 浓度为 25 μg/ml 的溶液。取溶液适量，置 1 cm 比色皿中，以蒸馏水做空白溶液，在 361 nm 波长下测定吸光度，计算维生素 B_{12} 的标示百分含量。

97

计算公式：

$$维生素 B_{12} 注射液标示百分含量 = \frac{\dfrac{A}{E_{1cm}^{1\%}} \times \dfrac{1}{100} \times D}{标示量（g/ml）} \times 100\%$$

$$E_{1cm}^{1\%}(361nm) = 207$$

式中，D 为稀释倍数。

五、注意事项

1. 比色皿应成对使用，不能随意调换。

2. 仪器使用前应开机预热，在不测定时，应随时打开暗箱盖，以保护光电管。

3. 比色皿一般用水振荡清洗，不能用毛刷刷洗，以免损伤比色皿。如比色皿被有机物沾污，可用 HCl－乙醇（1:2）浸泡片刻，再用水冲洗，不能用碱液或强氧化性洗液清洗。

4. 测定前，应用待测溶液润洗比色皿 2～3 次。比色皿内所盛待测溶液应超过皿高的 2/3 但不宜过满，否则溶液可能溢出，损坏仪器。使用后应立即将比色皿取出，用自来水及蒸馏水洗净，倒立晾干。

六、思考

制剂的含量为什么不能用百分含量表示？

Experiment 22　Determination of Vitamin B$_{12}$ Injection by UV Spectrophotometry

1. Objective

1.1　Master the method of drawing absorption curve and the principle of wavelength choosing.

1.2　Master the use of UV spectrophotometer and notes.

1.3　Master the determination of component content with the absorption coefficient method.

2. Principle

Absorption curve, also called absorption spectrum, is a curve drawn by taking the wavelength λ (nm) as the abscissa and the absorbance A (or the light transmittance T) as the ordinate. When establishing UV spectrophotometry for the determination of content, the absorption curve of the substance should first be drawn. The max absorption wavelength of the absorption spectrum of the target is usually selected as detection wavelength to improve the sensitivity and reduce the measurement error. If the target has several absorption peaks, the higher absorption peak without other substances interference is optional. Generally, the short wavelength end of the spectrum is not chosen as detection wavelength. In this experiment, the absorption curve of vitamin B$_{12}$ is drawn by continuous changing the detection wavelength of spectrophotometer.

There are serval methods including absorption coefficient method, working curve method and control method to determine the content of single-component sample. In this experiment, absorption coefficient method is used to determine the content of vitamin B$_{12}$ injection. Vitamin B$_{12}$ injection is pink to red liquid due to the cobalt contained in the molecular structure. Vitamin B$_{12}$ has three absorption peaks at 278 nm, 361 nm and 550 nm, respectively. Among them, the absorption peak at 361 nm is the highest with less interference. Therefore, the absorption coefficient at 361 nm ($E_{1cm}^{1\%} = 207$) can be used to calculate the content marked.

3. Apparatus and Materials

Apparatus: UV spectrophotometer, volumetric flask (10 ml), pipette (1 ml).

Materials: vitamin B$_{12}$ aqueous solution (0.1 mg/ml), vitamin B$_{12}$ injection.

4. Procedures

4.1 Drawing adsorption curve of vitamin B$_{12}$

Take appropriate amount of 0.1 mg/ml vitamin B$_{12}$ solution into 1 cm colorimetric ware and select distilled water as a blank solution to measure the absorbance in the 340~580 nm range. Among them, 340~370 nm and 540~580 nm are measured every 5 nm and the rest are measured every 20 nm. The absorption curve is drawn via the wavelength as abscissa, and absorbance as the vertical axis.

4.2 Determination of the content of vitamin B$_{12}$ injection

Pipet proper amount vitamin B$_{12}$ injection, dilute to 25 μg/ml solution with distilled water. Put the solution in 1 cm colorimetric ware and select distilled water as blank solution, then measure the absorbance at 361 nm, calculate the percentage content of vitamin B$_{12}$ using the following formula.

$$\text{Marked percentage of } V_{B_{12}} = \frac{\dfrac{A}{E_{1cm}^{1\%}} \times \dfrac{1}{100} \times D}{\text{Labeled amount（g/ml）}} \times 100\%$$

$$E_{1cm}^{1\%}(361nm) = 207$$

Notes: D is dilution factor.

5. Notes

5.1　The colorimetric wares should be used in pairs, and cannot exchange freely.

5.2　The spectrophotometer should be pretreatment before use, and when not measured, the lid should be opened to protect the photocell.

5.3　The colorimetric ware is generally washed with water, and cannot be brushed with a brush which will damage the colorimetric ware. If the colorimetric ware is contaminated with organic matter, it can be soaked in HCl-ethanol (1:2) for a while, and then rinsed with water. It cannot be washed with lye or strong oxidizing lotion.

5.4　The colorimetric ware should be rinsed for 2~3 times with the solution to be tested before the test. The solution in the colorimetric ware should be more than 2/3 of the height of colorimetric ware, but not over full; otherwise, the solution may overflow and damage the instrument. Remove the colorimetric ware immediately after use, and wash with tap water and distilled water, then dry upside down.

6. Questions

Why the content of formulations cannot be expressed as a percentage?

实验二十三　比色法测定芦丁的含量

一、实验目的

1. 掌握比色法的原理和操作方法。
2. 掌握标准曲线法测定含量的原理和方法。

二、实验原理

比色法是通过比较或测量有色物质溶液颜色深度来确定待测组分含量的方法。光电比色法是借助光电比色计来测量一系列标准溶液的吸光度，绘制标准曲线，然后根据被测试液的吸光度，从标准曲线上求出被测物质的含量的方法。其原理是基于被测物质溶液的颜色或加入显色剂后生成的有色溶液的颜色，其深度和物质含量成正比，则根据光被有色溶液吸收的强度，即可测定溶液中物质的含量。比色法测定前常需加入显色剂进行显色反应，显色反应须具良好的重现性与灵敏度。因此反应的条件必须严格控制：包括溶剂种类、试剂用量、溶液酸碱度、反应时间和比色时间等。

芦丁属于黄酮类化合物，其在中性或弱碱性及亚硝酸钠存在条件下与铝盐生成螯和物，加入氢氧化钠溶液后显红橙色，在约 500 nm 波长处有吸收峰且符合比尔定律，因此可采用比色法测定其含量。

三、仪器和材料

仪器　可见一紫外分光光度计，容量瓶（10 ml），移液管（5 ml）。
材料　芦丁标准品，亚硝酸钠试液，硝酸铝试液，氢氧化钠试液，乙醇（30%，60%）。

四、实验步骤

1. 0.1 mg/ml 芦丁标准溶液的配制　取 120℃真空干燥至恒重的芦丁标准品 20.0 mg，精密称定，置 100 ml 容量瓶中，加 60%乙醇适量使其溶解，并用 60%乙醇稀释至刻度，摇匀。精密吸取该溶液 25 ml，置 50 ml 容量瓶中，加蒸馏水至刻度，摇匀，即得。

2. 芦丁标准曲线的绘制　精密吸取 0.1 mg/ml 芦丁标准溶液 0.0 ml、1.0 ml、2.0 ml、3.0 ml、4.0 ml 及 5.0 ml，分别置 6 个 10 ml 容量瓶中，各加 30%乙醇使成 5.0 ml，各精密加入亚硝酸钠溶液（1:20）0.1 ml，摇匀，放置 6 min。再加硝酸铝溶液（1:10）0.5 ml，摇匀，再放置 6 min，加入氢氧化钠试液 4 ml，并用蒸馏水稀释至刻度，摇匀，放置 15 min。以不含芦丁的溶液作空白，在 510 nm 波长下测定各瓶溶液的吸收度。以芦丁浓度为横坐标，吸收度为纵坐标，绘制标准曲线。

3. 芦丁样品的测定　精密称取芦丁样品粉末约 20 mg，置 100 ml 容量瓶中，加 60%乙醇适量溶解并用 60%乙醇至刻度，摇匀。精密吸取此液 25 ml，置于 50 ml 容量瓶中，用蒸馏水稀释至刻度，摇匀。精密吸取上述溶液 3 ml，置于 10 ml 容量瓶中，照标准曲线的绘制项下的方法，自"加 30%乙醇使成 5.0 ml"起，依法操作并测定吸收度，从标准曲线中读出试样中无水芦丁的含量，并计算芦丁样品的含量：

$$\text{芦丁样品}\% = \frac{C_x \times D}{W} \times 100\%$$

式中，D 为稀释倍数。

五、注意事项

1. 实验中应注意平行原则，以减小操作误差。
2. 测定各标准溶液的吸收度时，一定要遵循先稀后浓的原则，减小测定误差。

六、思考

工作曲线法、吸收系数法和对照法各适用何种情况？

Experiment 23　Determination of the Content of Rutin by Colorimetry

1. Objective

1.1　Master the principle and operation of colorimetry.

1.2　Master the principle and method of content determination by standard curve method.

2. Principle

Colorimetric method is to determine the content of the target by comparing or measuring the color of the target solution. Photoelectric colorimetric method is to measure the absorbance of a series of standard solution using of photoelectric colorimeter, draw the standard curve, and then determine the content of the test substance based on the absorbance of the test solution in the standard curve. The principle is based on the color of the target itself or the color produced by color developing agent. The color depth is proportional to the content of the substance. So the content of the substance in the solution can be determined according to the intensity of the light absorbed by the colored solution. In colorimetric assay, color developing agent is usually needed to add to develop color. Color reaction must be good reproducibility and sensitivity, therefore, the reaction conditions including the type of solvent, reagents, pH, reaction time and colorimetric time, etc., must be strictly controlled.

Rutin belongs to the class of flavonoids, and it can generate chelates with aluminum salts in the presence of sodium nitrite in neutral or weakly basic condition. After addition of sodium hydroxide solution the solution becomes red-orange and has an absorption peak at about 500 nm. The adsorption follows Beer's law, so colorimetry can be used to determine the content of rutin.

3. Apparatus and Materials

Apparatus: UV spectrophotometer, volumetric flask (10 ml), pipette (5 ml).

Materials: Rutin standard, Sodium nitrite solution, Aluminum nitrate solution, Sodium hydroxide solution, Ethanol (30%, 60%).

4. Procedures

4.1　Preparation of 0.1 mg/ml rutin standard solution

Accurately weigh 20.0 mg rutin standard, which has been dried to a constant weight at 120 ℃ in advance, to 100 ml volumetric flask, and dissolve it in 60% ethanol followed by diluting with 60% ethanol to the mark, and shake well. Pipet 25 ml of above solution to 50 ml volumetric flask, and then add distilled water to the mark and shake well.

4.2 Drawing of rutin standard curve

Pipet 0.0 ml, 1.0 ml, 2.0 ml, 3.0 ml, 4.0 ml and 5.0 ml of 0.1 mg/ml standard solution of rutin to six 10 ml volumetric flasks, respectively, and dilute to 5.0 ml with 30% ethanol. Add 0.4 ml of sodium nitrite solution (1:20), shake well and allow to stand for 6 minutes. Then add 0.5 ml of aluminum nitrate solution (1:10), shake well, and then place for 6 minutes. Finally, add 4 ml of sodium hydroxide solution and dilute to the mark with distilled water. Shake well and allow standing for 15 minutes. The absorbance of each solution is measured at 510 nm using rutin-free solution as a blank. The standard curve is drawn with rutin concentration as abscissa and absorbance as ordinate.

4.3 Determination of rutin sample

20 mg of rutin sample powder is precisely weighed and placed in 100 ml volumetric flask. It is dissolved and diluted with 60% ethanol to the mark, and shaken well. Pipet this solution 25 ml to 50 ml volumetric flask, and then the solution is diluted with distilled water and shaken well. Then, 3 ml of the above solution is placed in 10 ml volumetric flask, and the same process is done from "add 30% ethanol to 5.0 ml" according to the operation of drawing standard curve. The concentration is read from the standard curve based on the absorbance measured. The content of rutin samples can be calculated as following formula:

$$\text{Percentage of rutin} = \frac{C_x \times D}{W} \times 100\%$$

Nodes: D is dilution factor.

5. Notes

5.1 Operators should pay attention to parallel operation to reduce operational errors.

5.2 When determination of the absorption of the standard solution, the order of measurement should be from thin to thick in order to reduce the measurement error.

6. Questions

What cases are suitable for working curve method, the absorption coefficient method and the control method?

实验二十四　荧光分光光度法测定维生素 B$_2$的含量

一、实验目的

1. 掌握荧光光度法的原理和方法。
2. 学会日立 F-4600 荧光分光光度计的基本操作。

二、实验原理

荧光是物质分子通过吸收电磁辐射而被激发,然后又从激发态返回到基态时发射的光。在稀溶液中,荧光强度 F 与荧光物质的浓度 C 有如下关系:$F=2.3 K' I_0 ECl$,这里 K' 和 I_0 均为常数,则该方程可变为 $F= kC$,这是荧光光度法定量分析的依据。

维生素 B$_2$ 分子中有三个芳香环,具有平面刚性结构,因此它能够发射荧光。维生素 B$_2$ 水溶液在紫外光照射下,发出黄绿色荧光。当低浓度（0.1～2.0 μg/ml）,pH=6～7 时,维生素 B$_2$ 荧光强度与其溶液浓度呈线性关系,此时其激发波长和发射波长分别为 454 nm 和 535 nm,因此可以用荧光光谱法测定维生素 B$_2$ 的含量。

三、仪器和材料

仪器　Hitachi F-4600 荧光分光光度计,石英皿,容量瓶（50 ml）,移液管（5 ml）,烧杯,滴管。

材料　维生素 B$_2$ 标准贮备液,维生素 B$_2$ 片,HAc 溶液(0.03 mol/L)。

四、实验步骤

1. 溶液的配制

（1）10 mg/L 维生素 B$_2$ 标准储备液的配制　精密称量 10.0 mg 的维生素 B$_2$ 对照品,以 0.03 mol/L HAc 溶液稀释至 1 000 ml 即得。

（2）标准系列溶液的配制　取此储备液 0.2 ml、0.4 ml、0.6 ml、0.8 ml、1.0 ml 分别置 10 ml 的容量瓶中,以去离子水稀释至刻度,摇匀,分别得到浓度约为 0.02 mg/ml, 0.04 mg/ml, 0.06 mg/ml, 0.08 mg/ml, 0.1 mg/ml 的溶液,待测。

（3）供试品储备液的配制　取维生素 B$_2$ 片（5 mg/片）共 20 片,精密称定。置研钵中,研细,从中取出适量（约相当于维生素 B$_2$ 10 mg）,精密称定,并移至 1 000 ml 容量瓶,以 0.03 mol/L HAc 溶解,超声提取 10 min。冷至室温,用 0.03 mol/L HAc 稀释至刻度。将此混合液用 0.45 μm 滤膜滤过,弃去初滤液,接续滤液待用。

2. 激发光谱和荧光发射光谱的绘制　本内容是实验者用于选择分析最佳条件。移取维生素 B$_2$ 标准储备液 0.4 ml 置 10 ml 的容量瓶中,以去离子水稀释至刻度,摇匀,待用。设置激发波长 λ_{ex} 为 454 nm,在 400～600 nm 范围内扫描发射波长,记录发射强度与发射波长间的函数关系,便得到荧光发射光谱。或者在固定 535 nm 为发射波长,在 350～550 nm 范围内扫描激发波长,记录荧光发射强度和激发波长的关系曲线,便得到激发光谱。从激发光谱图上找出其最大激发波长 λ_{ex}。在此激发波长下，从荧光发射光谱上找出其最大荧光发射波长 λ_{em}。

3. 绘制工作曲线　以 H_2O 作为空白，测定各标准溶液的荧光强度 F_1, F_2, …… F_5。以标准溶液的荧光强度为纵坐标，以维生素 B_2 标准溶液浓度为横坐标，绘制工作曲线并求出回归方程。

4. 供试品的测定　取供试品储备液 0.50 ml 于 10 ml 的容量瓶中，稀释至刻度。在同样条件下，测定此溶液的荧光值，用回归方程或在工作曲线上求得其浓度，并求算出维生素 B_2 片剂的标示百分含量。

五、注意事项

荧光分析法的灵敏度非常高，所以要仔细的操作以得到准确的结果。

六、思考

1. 标准曲线为直线吗？如果不是，曲线从何处开始弯曲的？请解释原因。
2. 荧光光谱法中，怎样确定用于样品分析的 λ_{ex} 和 λ_{em}？

Experiment 24　Determination of Vitamin B$_2$ by Fluorescence Spectrometry

1. Objective

1.1　Master the principle and method of fluorescence spectrometry.
1.2　Learn the operation of Hitachi F-4600 fluorescence spectrophotometer.

2. Principle

Fluorescence is an analytical important emission process in which molecules are excited by absorption of a beam of electromagnetic radiation, then radiant emission occurs as the excited species return to the ground state.

If the absorbance of a fluorescent analyte is small, there is a linear relation between the concentration, C, of a fluorescent analyte and the intensity of emission, F, given by the equation $F = 2.3\ K'\ I_0 EC$, where K' and I_0 are constant. This equation is reduced to $F = kC$, which is the basis for quantitative methods based on fluorescence.

Vitamin B$_2$ can emit fluorescence, because its molecules have rigid structures that are often planar and have aromatic groups. The aqueous solution of vitamin B$_2$ can produce yellow-green fluorescence under ultraviolet light，and the intensity of fluorescence is proportional to the concentration of vitamin B$_2$ in its low concentration ($0.1 \sim 2.0$ μg/ml) at pH $6 \sim 7$. The fluorescence excitation wavelength is 454 nm, and the emission wavelength is 535 nm under the above conditions. So vitamin B$_2$ can be determined by fluorescence spectrometer.

3. Apparatus and Materials

Apparatus: Hitachi F-4600 Fluorescence Spectrometer, quartz cell, volumetric flask (50 ml), pipette (5 ml), beaker, dropper.
Materials: vitamin B$_2$ standard stock solution, vitamin B$_2$ tablets, 0.03 mol/L HAc solution.

4. Procedures

4.1　Preparation of solutions

4.1.1　Preparation of Vitamin B$_2$ standard stock solution
Weigh accurately 10 mg vitamin B$_2$ (reference substance), dissolve in 0.03 mol/L HAc solution, and dilute to 1000 ml.
4.1.2　Preparation of standard solutions

Transfer 0.2 ml, 0.4 ml, 0.6 ml, 0.8 ml, and 1.0 ml of Vitamin B_2 standard stock solution to separate 10 ml volumetric flasks. Dilute the contents of each flask with water to volume, and mix to obtain known vitamin B_2 concentrations of about 0.02 mg/ml, 0.04 mg/ml, 0.06 mg/ml, 0.08 mg/ml, and 0.1 mg/ml, respectively.

4.1.3   The preparation of sample stock solution

Weigh accurately 20 tablets (5 mg/tablet) and grind to fine powder in a mortar. Transfer an accurately weighed quantity of the powder equivalent to about 10 mg of vitamin B_2 to a 1000 ml volumetric flask, add 0.03 mol/L HAc solution, and sonicate for 10 min to dissolve. Cool to room temperature, and dilute with 0.03 mol/L HAc solution to volume. Filter the mixture through a membrane with a 0.45 μm, discarding the first few ml of the filtrate, and retain the filtrate for the analysis.

4.2   Plot the fluorescence excitation and emission spectra

This allows the experimenter to choose optimum conditions for the analysis. Transfer 0.4 ml vitamin B_2 standard stock solution to a 10 ml volumetric flask, dilute to the volume with water. If the excitation wavelength is fixed at one wavelength (454 nm) and the intensity is plotted as a function of the emission wavelength (400~600 nm), the result is called an emission spectrum. The other possibility is to fix the wavelength (535 nm) at which the fluorescence intensity is measured by varying the excitation wavelength (350~550 nm). This results in an excitation spectrum.

Record the excitation and emission spectra of the solution to determine the maxium wavelengths of excitation (λ_{ex}) and the emission (λ_{em}).

4.3   Preparation of the standard curve

Determine the fluorescence intensities (F_1, F_2, ... F_5) of the solutions against the blank. Plot the fluorescence intensities of the standard solutions versus the concentration of vitamin B_2, and draw the straight line and obtain a regression equation.

4.4   Determination of the sample solution

Transfer 0.5 ml sample stock solution to a 10 ml volumetric flask, dilute to volume with water. Measure the fluorescence intensity of the solutions. From the graph (or regression equation) obtained, determine the concentration (C) of vitamin B_2 in the sample solution.

Calculate the percentage of the labeled amount of vitamin B_2 in the portion of tablets.

5. Notes

The sensitivity of fluorescence spectrometry is very high, so we must carefully operate in order to get accurate results.

6. Questions

1. Is the standard curve a linear one? If not, where does it begin to bend? Explain the reason.
2. How to determine the λ_{ex} and λ_{em} of the sample for analysis in fluorescence spectrometry?

实验二十五　苯和二甲苯气相色谱实验条件的考察

一、实验目的

1. 掌握通过对比已知物的定性分析的原理和方法。
2. 掌握色谱图改变对实验数据的影响。
3. 学会气相色谱系统的操作。

二、实验原理

通过比较已知物的定性分析，根据同一种物质在相同色谱条件下保留值相同的原理。该方法用于在相同条件下分别测出已知物质和样品的色谱图，然后比较与对照品组成相同的组分作对照分析，或向样品中加入合适的已知物质，去比较加入前后色谱图的改变。如果经测定的组分的色谱峰相对增大了，则可初步确定两者具有相同的物质，该方法可适用于已知物质范围未知试样的分析。

根据中国药典，当测定药物的组成或通过色谱方法分析药物时，用规定的对照品进行试验和调节，使理论塔板数、分离度、对称因子满足最小值。如果不能满足要求，则通过改变色谱条件（如柱长、载体、填充柱）或分离条件（如柱温、载气的流速、进样体积、流动相的用量）来满足要求。

三、仪器和材料

仪器　岛津 GC – 2010 气相色谱仪，1.0 μl 微量注射器。

材料　甲醇（色谱纯），苯，甲苯以及苯和甲苯混合溶液。

四、实验步骤

1. 色谱条件

色谱柱：Rtx – 1 (30 m × 0.32 mm × 0.25 μm) 毛细管柱

柱温：100℃

检测器：氢火焰离子化检测器、检测器温度 150℃

气化室温度：150℃

载气流量：N_2, 30 ml/min；H_2, 40 ml/min；空气，500 ml/min

进样量：0.5 μl

分流比：1:30

2. 溶液配制

（1）对照溶液配制

苯对照溶液：精密量取 1 ml 苯，置于 100 ml 容量瓶中，用甲醇稀释至刻度，摇匀，密封，备用。

甲苯对照溶液：精密量取 1 ml 甲苯，置于 100 ml 容量瓶中，用甲醇稀释至刻度，摇匀，密封，备用。

（2）样品溶液的制备

稀释溶液：配制约每 100 ml 甲醇含 1 μl 苯和甲苯溶液，摇匀，密封，备用。

浓缩溶液：配制含 50% 苯和甲苯的混合溶液 10 ml，摇匀，密封，备用。

3. 测定 待基线平直后，分别取 0.5 μl 的苯、甲苯和稀释后的样品溶液，注入 GC（取平均值的 2 倍），得到色谱图，从图中读取各组分色谱峰的峰宽 W 和保留时间 t_R，样品中各峰的归属由各成分的保留值确定。将 0.5 μl 浓缩样品溶液进入 GC 中，并记录流出曲线。

测定每个峰的峰宽和保留时间，并用分离方程确定稀和浓溶液中的分离度。

$$R = \frac{2(t_{R_{methylbenzen}} - t_{R_{benzene}})}{W_{methybenzene} + W_{benzene}}$$

增加柱温，取 0.5 μl 稀溶液进入 GC，并且记录流出曲线，保留时间和峰宽，计算各组分的分离度。

升温前后，稀释液中各组分中保留时间和分离度的比较。

五、注意事项

1. 对标准样品的保留值进行定性分析时，应保证实验条件的一致性。有时由于色谱柱不合适，两种组分的位置恰好相同或相似。因此，应选择一种具有不同极性或其他类型的替代品来进一步确认。如果峰值仍然相同，两者都可以初步确定为同一物质。

2. 当色谱柱温度发生变化时，应该在柱温箱温度不变、基线稳定后再进行注入样品。

Experiment 25   Experimental Conditions Study for Benzene and Methylbenzene Analyzed by Gas Chromatography

1. Objective

1.1   Master the principles and methods of qualitative analysis by comparing known substance.

1.2   Master the impact of changes of chromatography conditions on the experimental data.

1.3   Learn the operation of gas chromatography system.

2. Principle

Qualitative analysis by comparing known substance is carried out on the principle that the same substance in the same column on the same operating conditions has the same retention value. The method is to measure the chromatogram of a known substance and the sample in the same experimental conditions, respectively, and then compare the retention value of the component to be identified to that of the reference substance to take a qualitative analysis; or add appropriate known substance to the sample, and compare the chromatogram change before and after the addition. If the peak of the identified component becomes relatively high, then it can be determined initially that both are the same substance. The method is applicable to the unknown samples within the scope of known substances.

According to the Chinese Pharmacopoeia, the equipment should be tested and adjusted using the required reference substance to meet the minimum number of theoretical plates, resolution and symmetry factor when determining drug contents or identifying drugs by chromatography. If it does not meet the requirements, it should be promoted by changing the column conditions (such as column length, performance of carrier, and performance of filling column, etc.) or the separation conditions (such as column temperature, carrier gas flow rate, liquid dosage, and injection volume, etc.) to meet the requirement.

3. Apparatus and Materials

Apparatus: SHIMADZU GC-2010 Gas Chromatograph (GC), 1.0 μl micro injector.

Materials: methanol (chromatographic grade), benzene, methylbenzene and a mixture solution of the two components.

4. Procedures

4.1 Experimental conditions

Chromatographic Column: Rtx-1(30 m × 0.32 mm×0.25 μm) capillary column.

Column temperature: 100 ℃.

Detector: FID, temperature 150 ℃.

Temperature of gasification room: 150 ℃.

Gas flow rate: N_2, 30 ml/min, H_2, 40 ml/min, atmosphere, 500 ml/min.

Injection volume: 0.5 μl.

Split ratio: 1:30.

4.2 Solution Preparation

4.2.1 Preparation of reference substance solution

Benzene reference solution: A precise volume of 1 ml benzene is taken, placed in 100 ml volumetric flask, diluted to scale with methanol, shaken, sealed, and ready for use.

Methylbenzene reference solution: A precise volume of 1 ml methylbenzene is taken, placed in a 100 ml volumetric flask, diluted to scale with methanol, shaken, sealed, and ready for use.

4.2.2 Preparation of sample solution

Diluted solution: Prepare about 100 ml methanol solution containing 1 μl of each benzene and methylbenzene in the flask, shake, sealed, and ready for use.

Concentrated solution: Prepare a mixture solution containing 50% of benzene and methylbenzene, respectively, in 10 ml flask, shake, sealed, and ready for use.

4.3 Determination

Samples benzene, methylbenzene and diluted solution is taken 0.5 μl, respectively, after the baseline being straight, and injected into the GC (take the average of 2 times). Draw the outflow curve, and record each component peak width w and the retention time t_R. The attribution of each peak in the sample was identified by the retention value of each component.

Take 0.5 μl concentrated sample solution into the GC, and record the outflow curve.

Measure each component of the peak width W and the retention time t_R of concentrated solution, and determine the separation R of benzene and methylbenzene in dilute and concentrated solution using the following equation.

$$R = \frac{2(t_{R_{methylbenzen}} - t_{R_{benzene}})}{W_{methybenzene} + W_{benzene}}$$

Increase the column temperature, and take 0.5 μl diluted solution into the GC, and record the outflow curve, as well as the retention time and peak width, and calculate the separation of each component.

Compare the changes of retention time and resolution of each component in diluted solution before and after warming up.

5. Notes

5.1　When qualitative analysis was done by comparing with the retention value of standard sample, the consistency of experimental conditions should be ensured. Sometimes the position of two different components happened to be the same or similar due to the unsuitable chromatography column. So, an alternative one with different polar or of other type should be chosen to further confirm. If the peak is still the same, both can be initially determined to be the same substance.

5.2　When the column temperature was changed, another injection should be performed after the temperature column box temperature being constant and the baseline being stable.

实验二十六　HPLC 法测定感冒胶囊中咖啡因的含量

一、实验目的

1. 掌握高效液相色谱仪的原理和使用方法。
2. 掌握外标标准曲线定量方法。
3. 熟悉反相色谱的原理和应用。

二、实验原理

复方感冒胶囊由对乙酰氨基酚、阿司匹林和咖啡因等组成，其中咖啡因具有兴奋中枢神经、扩张血管等生物活性，与对乙酰氨基酚合用，能增强镇痛作用。测定咖啡因的方法有薄层层析法、分光光度法、气相色谱法等多种方法。本实验采用反相高效液相色谱法，以甲醇–水（35:65）作流动相，以 275 nm 为检测波长，测定常用复方感冒药中的咖啡因含量，其中的对乙酰氨基酚等组分可与咖啡因很好分离。本方法灵敏、快速、准确可靠，可用于复方制剂的质量控制。

三、仪器和材料

仪器　高效液相色谱仪，ODS 柱，容量瓶（100 ml），容量瓶（50 ml），移液管（体积 5 ml），微量注射器，研钵，漏斗。

材料　咖啡因对照品，1 g/L 咖啡因标准储备溶液（将咖啡因于 110℃下烘干 1 小时，准确称取 0.1 g，用重蒸水溶解并定容于 100 ml 容量瓶中，则标准储备液浓度为 1 g/L），甲醇（色谱纯），复方感冒胶囊，二次重蒸馏水。

四、实验步骤

1. 流动相的配制　分别量取 70 ml 甲醇和 130 ml 二次重蒸馏水，混匀。用微孔滤膜过滤，超声脱气备用。

2. 色谱条件　流动相：甲醇–水（35:65）；流速：1 ml/min；检测波长 275 nm；色谱柱：C_{18} 柱。

3. 工作曲线的制作　分别量取 1.00 ml、2.00 ml、3.00 ml、4.00 ml、5.00 ml 咖啡因标准储备液转移至 50 ml 容量瓶中，加蒸馏水定容至刻度，摇匀，则其浓度分别为 20.0 mg/L、40.0 mg/L、60.0 mg/L、80.0 mg/L、100.0 mg/L。调整仪器待基线平稳后，各进样 20 μl 溶液，得到色谱流出曲线，记录峰面积。以咖啡因浓度（mg/L）为横坐标，以峰面积为纵坐标绘制工作曲线，得到回归方程 Y=a+bX 和线性回归系数 r。

4. 样品的测定　取 20 粒感冒胶囊，倾出内容物称重，求出平均粒重。准确称取一定量的粉末（约含咖啡因 15 mg）至 50 ml 容量瓶中，用重蒸馏水定容至刻度，摇匀，过滤，取续滤液 5 ml 转移至 50 ml 容量瓶中，用重蒸馏水定容至刻度，摇匀，微孔滤膜过滤，20 μl 进样。根据色谱峰面积，求出样品中咖啡因的含量(用标示量%表示)。

五、注意事项

1. 开机后需要平衡色谱系统半小时后再进样。
2. 流动相配制好后，一定要进行过滤和脱气。
3. 在换流动相之前应停泵。
4. 实验结束后需要用甲醇冲洗色谱柱。

六、思考

1. 用外标法定量的优缺点是什么？还可以采取何种定量方法？
2. 当室温发生变化时，保留值会如何变化？为什么？
3. 反相色谱法中，流动相 pH 应该控制在什么范围之内？

Experiment 26　Determination of Caffeine in Ganmao Capsule by HPLC

1. Objective

1.1　Master the principle and operation of HPLC.

1.2　Master the quantitative method of external standard curve.

1.3　Familiar with the principle and application of RP-HPLC.

2. Principle

Ganmao capsule consists of acetaminophen, aspirin, caffeine and so on. Caffeine has the biological activity of stimulating central nervous system and dilating blood vessels. It can be combined with acetaminophen to enhance analgesic effect. There are many methods to determine caffeine, such as TLC, spectrophotography, GC and so on. In this experiment, we will assay caffeine by high performance liquid chromatography with an ultraviolet detector at 275 nm. The column is C_{18} and the mobile phase consists of methanol-water (35:65, V/V). Acetaminophen and caffeine can be well separated. The method is sensitive, rapid, accurate and reliable, and can be used for quality control of compound preparation.

3. Apparatus and Materials

Apparatus: HPLC apparatus, ODS column, volumetric flask(50 ml), volumetric flask(100 ml), pipet(5 ml), micro syringe, mortar, funnel.

Materials: reference substance of caffeine, 1 g/L caffeine standard solution (Weigh accurately 0.1 g caffeine that has been previously dried for 1 h at a temperature of 110 ℃. Dissolve it in 100 ml redistilled water, and shake well), methanol (HPLC reagent), Ganmao Capsules, redistilled water.

4. Procedures

4.1　Preparation of mobile solution

The mobile phase is prepared by mixing 70 ml methanol and 130 ml redistilled water, then filtered by microporous membrane and then degassed by ultrasonic.

4.2　Chromatographic conditions

Mobile phase: methanol-water (35:65); Flow rate: 1 ml/min; Detecting Wavelength: 275 nm; Chromatographic column: C_{18}.

4.3　Preparation of standard curve

Pipet 1.00 ml, 2.00 ml, 3.00 ml, 4.00 ml and 5.00 ml of caffeine standard solution(1 g/L) into five 50 ml volumetric flasks, add distilled water to the line, mix well. Their concentrations are 20.0 mg/L, 40.0 mg/L, 60.0 mg/L, 80.0 mg/L, 100.0 mg/L, respectively. Adjust the instrument until the baseline is stable, and inject 20 μl solution into HPLC respectively. The chromatogram is obtained, and the peak area is recorded. We can draw regression curve with caffeine concentration as abscissa and the peak area as ordinate. At the same time, we can get the regression equation $Y = a + b X$ and regression coefficient r.

4.4　Sample determination

Weight 20 capsules after removing capsule shells, and calculate the average mass of drug power that a bolus holds. Accurately transfer a certain amount of powder (equivalent to about 15 mg of caffeine) to a 50 ml volumetric flask, add distilled water to volume, shake well and filter. Transfer 5 ml of continuous filtrate to a 50 ml volumetric flask, add distilled water to the line, mix well. Filter through microporous filter membrane. Inject 20 μl sample solution into HPLC. The concentration of caffeine can be calculated by peak area (expressed in % labeled amount).

5. Notes

5.1　The balance chromatographic system needs to be balanced for half an hour before the sample is injected.

5.2　Mobile phase should be filtered and degassed before use.

5.3　Stop the pump before changing mobile phase.

5.4　Rinse the column with methanol after the experiment is over.

6. Questions

1. What are the advantages and disadvantages of external standard method? What other quantitative methods can be used?

2. How does retention value change when the room temperature changes? Why?

3. What is the range of pH of mobile phase in reversed-phase chromatography?

实验二十七　水杨酸红外光谱的测定

一、实验目的

1. 掌握固体试样的制备方法。
2. 学习用红外光谱对化合物进行定性分析的方法。
3. 熟悉红外光谱仪的工作原理和操作方法。

二、实验原理

红外光谱定性分析，一般采用两种方法。

1. 已知标准物对照法　取标准试样和待测试样在完全相同的工作条件下，分别绘制出 IR 图谱进行对照，图谱相同，则为同一化合物。

2. 标准图谱查对法　标准图谱查对法是一种直接、可靠的方法。根据待测试样的来源、物理常数、分子式及图谱中的特征谱带，查对标准图谱来确定化合物。常用的标准图谱为萨特勒红外图谱集（The Sadtler Handbook of Infrared Spectra）。

三、仪器和材料

仪器　岛津 Irprestige-21 红外光谱仪，红外线灯，玛瑙研钵，压片模具。
材料　水杨酸（纯度大于 98%），KBr（光谱纯），石蜡油。

四、实验步骤

1. 压片法　取干燥的水杨酸试样约 2 mg 置于玛瑙研钵中，加入干燥的 KBr 粉末约 200 mg，充分磨细混匀（颗粒粒度约为 2 μm）。取出约 100 mg 混合物装入干净的压模内铺匀，置于压片机上压片（压力不超过 10 MPa），制成透明试样薄片。

2. 糊状法　取少量干燥样品置玛瑙研钵中，滴入几滴石蜡油，研磨至呈均匀的浆糊状，取此糊状物涂在空白 KBr 片上，即可测定。

3. 测定　将上述制备的样品置试样架上，插入红外光谱仪试样池的光路中，用纯 KBr 薄片为参比片，按仪器操作方法从 400 cm^{-1}～4 000 cm^{-1} 扫描，即得水杨酸的红外光谱图。从红外光谱中找出主要水杨酸吸收峰的归属记录在下表中（见表 27-1），并将扫描得到的图谱与已知标准谱进行对照比较。

表 27-1　水杨酸吸收峰的归属

归属	v_{O-H}	$v_{C=C}$	$v_{C=O}$	δ_{Ar-H}
峰位(cm^{-1})				

五、注意事项

1. 为避免受潮，制样应在红外线灯下进行。

2. 压片制样时，物料必须磨细并混合均匀，加入到模具中需均匀平整，否则不易获得均匀透明的试样。

3. 扫描结束后，取下试样架，取出薄片，务必将模具、试样架、研钵等用乙醇擦净晾干。

六、思考

红外光谱法对固体试样的制片有什么要求？

Experiment 27　Determination of Salicylic Acid Chemical Structure by IR Spectrophotometry

1. Objective

1.1　Master the preparation of solid sample.

1.2　Study on qualitative analysis of compounds by infrared spectroscopy.

1.3　Familiar with the working principle and operation method of infrared spectrometer.

2. Principle

There are two qualitative analysis methods to identify drug by IR.

2.1　Comparison with known standard

Plot the IR spectrum of standard sample and tested sample under the same work condition, respectively. The IR spectrum of tested sample comparing with the one of the standard sample, if IR spectrums are the same, they are the same compounds.

2.2　Comparison with standard atlas

This method is direct and reliable. According to the source, physical constants, molecular formula, characteristic band of the sample, you can compare the atlas with standard atlas to identify the compound. The most commonly used standard atlas is the Sadtler Handbook of Infrared Spectra.

3. Apparatus and Materials

Apparatus: Shimadzu Irprestige-21 infrared spectrophotometer, infrared lamp, agate mortar，compression mold.

Materials: salicylic acid（the purity is more than 98%）, potassium bromide(spectrum reagent), liquid paraffin.

4. Procedures

4.1　Pressing method

Weigh 2 mg dry sample, mix it with 200 mg KBr（spectrum reagent）in an agate mortar and triturate the mixture under infrared lamp（the granularity of the particle is about 2 μm）. Remove about 100 mg mixture into compression mold, distribute it well, and place it on the pressure machine to make a transparent sample sheet.

4.2　Paste method

A small amount of dry samples are placed in agate mortar, and a few drops of paraffin oil are dripped into the mortar, then ground to a uniform paste. The paste is coated on a blank KBr sheet and could be determined.

4.3 Determination

The sample prepared above is placed on the sample holder, pure KBr slice is used as a reference sheet. According to the instrument operation method, scan from 400 cm^{-1} to 4000 cm^{-1} and plot the IR spectrum. Find out the absorption frequency of the primary functional group of salicylic acid and record in the following table (Table 27-1) , and compare with the standard atlas.

Table 27-1   The absorption frequency of salicylic acid

adscription	ν_{O-H}	$\nu_{C=C}$	$\nu_{C=O}$	δ_{Ar-H}
peak position (cm^{-1})				

5. Notes

5.1   Triturate the sample under infrared lamp to avoid moisture absorption.

5.2   When the sample is prepared by pressing method, the material must be grinded and mixed evenly, well-distributed in the mold. Otherwise, it is not easy to obtain uniform and transparent samples.

5.3   After scanning, take down the sample holder, take out of the slice, be sure to clean the mold, sample holder and mortar with alcohol.

6. Questions

What kind of solid sample can be used to plot IR spectrum?

实验二十八　薄层色谱的制备和应用

一、实验目的

1. 了解薄层色谱的基本原理和应用。
2. 掌握薄层色谱的操作技术。

二、实验原理

薄层色谱（thin layer chromatography）常用 TLC 表示，又称薄层层析，属于固−液吸附色谱。样品在薄层板上的吸附剂（固定相）和溶剂（流动相）之间进行分离。由于各种化合物的吸附能力各不相同，在展开剂上移时，它们进行不同程度的解吸，从而达到分离的目的。

被分离物质如果是有色组分，展开后薄层色谱板上即呈现出有色斑点。如果化合物本身无色，则可用碘蒸气熏的方法显色。还可使用腐蚀性的显色剂如浓硫酸、浓盐酸和浓磷酸等。对于含有荧光剂的薄层板在紫外光下观察，展开后的有机化合物在亮的荧光背景上呈暗色斑点。

薄层色谱的吸附剂最常用的是氧化铝和硅胶。硅胶吸附剂分为两种：含煅石膏黏合剂的为硅胶 G；不含黏合剂的为硅胶 H。其颗粒大小一般为 260 目以上。颗粒太大，展开剂移动速度快，分离效果不好；反之，颗粒太小，溶剂移动太慢，斑点不集中，效果也不理想。

薄层板制备的好坏直接影响色谱的结果。薄层应尽量均匀且厚度要固定。否则，在展开时前沿不齐，色谱结果也不易重复。将涂布好的薄层板置于室温晾干后，还需放在烘箱内加热活化，活化条件根据需要而定。硅胶板一般在烘箱中渐渐升温，维持（105～110）℃活化 30 分钟。氧化铝板在 200℃烘 4 小时可得到活性为Ⅱ级的薄板，在（150～160）℃烘 4 小时可得活性为Ⅲ～Ⅳ级的薄板。活化后的薄层板放在干燥器内保存待用。薄层色谱的用途如下。

1. 化合物的定性检验　（通过与已知标准物对比的方法进行未知物的鉴定）在条件完全一致的情况，纯化合物在薄层色谱中呈现一定的移动距离，称比移值（R_f 值），所以利用薄层色谱法可以鉴定化合物的纯度或确定两种性质相似的化合物是否为同一物质。但影响比移值的因素很多，如薄层的厚度，吸附剂颗粒的大小，酸碱性，活性等级，外界温度和展开剂纯度、组成、挥发性等。所以，要获得重现的比移值就比较困难。为此，在测定某一试样时，最好用已知样品进行对照。

$$R_f = \frac{\text{溶质最高浓度中心至原点中心的距离}}{\text{溶剂前沿至原点中心的距离}}$$

2. 快速分离少量物质　几到几十微克，甚至 0.01 μg。

3. 跟踪反应进程　在进行化学反应时，常利用薄层色谱观察原料斑点的逐步消失，来判断反应是否完成。

4. 化合物纯度的检验　只出现一个斑点，且无拖尾现象，为纯物质。

三、仪器和材料

仪器　载玻片，层析缸，烘箱。

材料　硅胶 G，羧甲基纤维素钠水溶液（0.5%），槐花粉，甲醇。

四、实验步骤

1. 薄层板的制备　在研钵中放入 4 g 硅胶 G，加入（10～12）ml 0.5% 的羧甲基纤维素钠水溶液，研磨，调成糊状。将配制好的浆料用药匙舀到清洁干燥的载玻片上，使其表面均匀平滑，在室温下晾干后，烘箱内（105～110℃）恒温活化半小时。每人两片。

2. 药材试样的制备　取槐花粉末 0.2 g，加甲醇 5 ml，密塞，超声 10 min，放置 10 min，滤过，滤液作为供试品溶液。

3. 对照品溶液的制备　称取一定芦丁和槲皮素对照品，制成甲醇溶液，作为对照品溶液。

4. 点板　用铅笔轻轻画出一条平行于玻璃板底边的细线，并间隔 1 cm 用铅笔轻点作为点板标记。用毛细管蘸取试样溶液和对照品溶液，分别在同一块薄层板上点样。

5. 展开　吹干样点，竖直放入盛有展开剂（乙酸乙酯－甲酸－水 8:1:1）的有盖展开槽中。展开剂要接触到吸附剂下沿，但切勿接触到样点。盖上盖子，展开。待展开剂上行到距上沿 1 cm 时，取出薄层板，画出展开剂的前沿线。

6. 显色　挥发干展开剂，置紫外光灯（365 nm）下检视，再用三氯化铝试液显色后在紫外灯下观察现象。

五、注意事项

1. 载玻片应干净且不被手污染，吸附剂在载玻片上应均匀平整。

2. 点样不能戳破薄层板面，各样点间距 1～1.5 cm，样点直径应不超过 2 mm。若样品溶液太稀，可重复点样，但应待前次点样的溶剂挥发后方可重新点样，以防样点过大，造成拖尾、扩散等现象，而影响分离效果。

3. 展开时，不要让展开剂前沿上升至底线。否则，无法确定展开剂上升高度，即无法求得 R_f 值和准确判断粗产物中各组分在薄层板上的相对位置。

六、思考

1. 如何利用 R_f 值来鉴定化合物？
2. 薄层色谱法点样应注意些什么？
3. 常用的薄层色谱的显色剂是什么？

Experiment 28　Preparation and Application of Thin Layer Chromatography

1. Objective

1.1　Learn the basic principles and applications of TLC.

1.2　Master the operation of thin-layer chromatography.

2. Principle

Thin Layer Chromatography abbreviated as TLC belongs to solid-liquid adsorption chromatography. The sample is separated between the adsorbent (stationary phase) on the TLC plate and the solvent (mobile phase). Due to the different adsorption capacities of various compounds, they are desorbed to different extents when the developer moves up, thereby achieving the purpose of separation.

If the material to be separated is a colored component, the developed TLC will show colored spots. If the compound itself is colorless, iodine vapor may be used to develop color. Corrosive developers such as concentrated sulfuric acid, concentrated hydrochloric acid and concentrated phosphoric acid may also be used. For thin-layer plates containing fluoresces observed under UV light, the separated organic compounds appear dark spots on a bright fluorescent background.

The most commonly used adsorbents for thin-layer chromatography are alumina and silica gel. Silica gel adsorbent is divided into two kinds: Silica gel H: No adhesive; Silica gel G: With Calcined gypsum. The particle size is generally less than 260 meshes. Developers move fast with too large particles lead to poor separation; On the other hand, the solvent moves too slowly with too small particles, the spots are not concentrated and the result is not satisfactory.

The quality of prepared TLC plates directly affects the results of chromatography. Thin layer should be uniform and the thickness should be fixed. Otherwise, the forefront is irregular and the chromatographic results are not easy to repeat. After a good coated TLC plate left at room temperature drying, activated in an oven heat, activation conditions in accordance with needs. Usually silica gel plates in an oven gradually warming, maintained the activation of $105\sim110$ ℃ for 30 min. While 4 h available alumina plate bake at 200 ℃ obtain Ⅱ grade sheets activity, bake at $150\sim160$ ℃ for 4 h to obtain a thin plate Ⅲ-Ⅳ activity level. The activated lamina stored in a desiccator until use.

Application of TLC as follows.

2.1 Qualitative test of compounds. (Identification of unknowns by a method of comparison with known standards)

In the case of exactly the same conditions, pure compounds in the TLC show a certain distance of movement, known as the ratio (R_f value), so the use of thin-layer chromatography can be identified compounds purity or to determine whether two compounds of similar nature are the same substance. However, there are many factors affecting the specific value of the shift, such as the thickness of the thin layer, the size of the adsorbent particles, acid-base, activity level, external temperature and developer purity, composition, volatility and the like. Therefore, it is more difficult to obtain the reproduced ratio value. For this reason, in the determination of a sample, it is best to use known samples for control.

$$R_f = \frac{\text{Distance between the origin center to the spot center}}{\text{Distance between the origin centerto the solvent front}}$$

2.2 Rapid separation of a small amount of material. (A few to tens of micrograms, or even 0.01 mg)

2.3 Track the progress of the reaction. In the chemical reaction, often using thin layer chromatography to observe the gradual disappearance of raw material spots to determine whether the reaction is completed.

2.4 The purity of the test compound (appears only one spot, and no tailing, as a pure substance.)

3. Apparatus and Materials

Apparatus: slide, oven, expansion tank.

Materials: Silica gel G, aqueous solution of sodium carboxymethyl (0.5%), Sophora japonicus, methanol.

4. Procedures

4.1 Preparation of thin layer plate

In a mortar, 4 g of silica gel G was added, and (10~12) ml of a 0.5% aqueous solution of sodium carboxymethyl cellulose was added thereto, followed by grinding and stirring into a paste. Pour the prepared slurry onto a clean, dry slide with a spoon to make the surface smooth and uniform, and then dry it at room temperature. Activate at (105~110) ℃ for half an hour. (Two slides per person).

4.2 Preparation of medicinal samples

Take *Sophora japonicus* powder 0.2 g into a test tube, add 5 ml of methanol plug ultrasonic 10 min and place 10 min, then filter and take the filtrate as the test solution.

4.3 Preparation of reference solution

Weigh a certain amount of rutin and quercetin reference substance, made of methanol solution, as a reference solution.

4.4　Spotting

Gently draw a fine line parallel to the bottom edge of the glass sheet with a pencil and draw points with 1 cm intervals as markings. Dip the sample solution and the reference solution by capillary and spot onto the TLC plate.

4.5　Chromatography

Dry sample point and put the plate vertically into the expansion tank containing the developing solvent (ethyl acetate-formic acid-water 8:1:1). The developing agent shall be in contact with the lower edge of the adsorbent, but do not touch the sample. Cover the lid and chromatograph. When the agent up to 1 cm from the upper edge. Remove the plate and draw the front of the developer.

4.6　Coloring

Dry developing agent and observe under ultraviolet light (365 nm). Then color with aluminum chloride solution and observe again under ultraviolet light (365 nm).

5. Notes

5.1　Slides should be clean and not be contaminated by hands; adsorbent on the slide should be smooth.

5.2　Point can not puncture the surface of the plate. It can be repeated spotting if the sample solution is too thin, but the sample should not be spotted until the solvent volatilizes to prevent too large spot, resulting in tailing, spreading and other phenomena, and affect the separation effect.

5.3　Do not let the forefront of the developer rise to the top. Otherwise, it is not possible to determine the rising height of the developer. It means that it is unable to obtain the R_f value and accurately determine the relative position of each component in the crude product on the TLC plate.

6. Questions

6.1　How to identify compounds by R_f value?

6.2　What should be noted when pointing?

6.3　What is the commonly used TLC color-developing agent?

第三部分　设计性实验

实验二十九　食醋总酸度的测定

一、实验目的

1. 学习实样滴定分析的基本方法和基本过程。
2. 掌握碱标准溶液配制和标定的方法。
3. 掌握食醋总酸度的测定原理、方法和操作技术。

二、实验内容

1. 设计用滴定分析法测定市售食醋总酸度的实验方案，并简述实验原理。
2. 根据设计的实验方案选择实验试剂和仪器。
3. 根据拟定的实验方案进行滴定分析，注意标准溶液的配制和标定。
4. 按前面学过的分析记录格式做表格，记录数据并进行数据计算处理。市售食醋总酸度以"100 ml 食醋中含醋酸的质量（g/100 ml）"表示。

三、提示

1. 食醋中的酸性物质主要是醋酸。
2. 食醋样品需经稀释才能进行滴定分析。
3. 食醋的颜色会影响滴定终点的颜色判断，可以选用活性炭脱色，但会造成测定结果偏低。
4. NaOH 标准溶液滴定醋酸，属强碱滴定弱酸，CO_2 的影响严重，注意除去所用蒸馏水中的 CO_2。

四、思考

1. 为什么食醋样品需经稀释才能进行滴定分析？
2. 如何去除实验用水中的 CO_2？
3. 如果滴定终点没有控制好，即 NaOH 标准溶液滴加过量，溶液显红色，有没有补救的办法？

Experiment 29　Determination of Total Acidity of Vinegar

1. Objective

1.1　Learn the method and process of titration analysis.

1.2　Master the methods of preparation and calibration of alkali standard solution.

1.3　Master the methods and operating techniques of determination of total vinegar acidity.

2. Experimental Content

2.1　Design the experimental program of titration analysis of the total acidity of commercially available vinegar, and describe the experimental principle briefly.

2.2　According to the experimental program designed to choose experimental reagents and apparatus.

2.3　Titrate according to the proposed experimental program, pay attention to preparation and calibration of the alkali standard solution.

2.4　Design the form to record the original data, and then data processing. The total acidity of vinegar is expressed as "acetate content (g/100 ml) in 100 ml vinegar".

3. Prompt

3.1　Acetic acid is the main acid in vinegar.

3.2　Vinegar samples need to be diluted for titration analysis.

3.3　The color of vinegar samples can affect the color judgment of the end point. You can bleach the color of vinegar samples using activated carbon, but it can result in low measurement results.

3.4　When acetic acid is titrated with NaOH standard solution as titrant, CO_2 can seriously affect the measurement results. Therefore, the removal of CO_2 in water is very necessary.

4. Questions

4.1　Why vinegar samples need to be diluted for titration analysis?

4.2　How to remove CO_2 in experimental water?

4.3　If the end point of titration is not controlled well, that is, NaOH standard solution dropping excess and the solution is red, is there any remedy?

实验三十 蛋壳中钙、镁的含量测定

一、实验目的

1. 学习用所学滴定知识解决实际问题的方法，提高分析问题、解决问题的能力。
2. 掌握滴定分析方法和操作技术。
3. 掌握滴定分析测定蛋壳中钙、镁含量的原理和方法。

二、实验内容

1. 设计用滴定分析法测定蛋壳中钙、镁含量的实验方案，并简述实验原理。
2. 根据设计的实验方案选择实验试剂和仪器。
3. 根据拟定的实验方案进行滴定分析，注意标准溶液的配制和标定。
4. 按前面学过的分析记录格式做表格，记录数据并进行数据计算处理。蛋壳中的钙、镁总量以 CaO 的质量百分含量表示。

三、提示

1. 蛋壳的主要成分为 $CaCO_3$，其次为 $MgCO_3$、蛋白质、色素及少量铁和铝元素。
2. 先粗略确定蛋壳粉中钙、镁含量，再估算蛋壳粉的称量范围。
3. 通常蛋壳中的钙、镁需要经过稀酸加热溶解转换为离子形式才能进行滴定分析。若试样中有不溶物（如蛋白质等）不影响测定。
4. 由于有蛋白质的存在，样品液定容时会产生少量泡沫。可以用蘸取了少量乙醇的玻璃棒轻触泡沫达到消泡的效果。
5. 可以分别用以下三种滴定分析法测定蛋壳中的钙、镁含量。
（1）EDTA 配位滴定法 蛋壳中钙、镁的含量测定可采用 EDTA 滴定法，在 pH = 10 的缓冲溶液中，以铬黑 T 为指示剂，EDTA 标准溶液为滴定剂进行测定。为提高配位选择性，滴定前加入掩蔽剂三乙醇胺，排除 Fe^{3+}、Al^{3+} 等离子对 Ca^{2+}、Mg^{2+} 离子测量的干扰。
（2）酸碱滴定法 蛋壳中碳酸盐能与盐酸发生反应，过量的盐酸可用 NaOH 标准溶液返滴。根据与 $CaCO_3$ 反应的盐酸的量求得蛋壳中钙、镁的含量。
（3）高锰酸钾滴定法 将蛋壳中钙、镁元素转变为离子形式，并与草酸形成难溶的草酸盐沉淀，过滤洗涤后将沉淀在酸液中溶解，然后用高锰酸钾标准溶液滴定与钙、镁离子结合的 $C_2O_4^{2-}$ 的含量，换算出蛋壳中钙、镁的含量。

四、思考

1. 如何确定蛋壳粉末的称量范围？
2. 蛋壳粉溶解稀释时为什么会出现泡沫？应如何消除泡沫？

Experiment 30   Determination of Calcium and Magnesium Content in Eggshell

1. Objective

1.1   Learn to use the titration knowledge to solve the practical problems, improving the ability to analyze and solve problems.

1.2   Master titration methods and operating techniques.

1.3   Master the principle and method of determination calcium and magnesium content in eggshell by titration analysis.

2. Experimental Content

2.1   Design the method of determination of calcium and magnesium content in eggshell by titration analysis, and describe the experimental principles briefly.

2.2   According to the experimental program designed to choose experimental reagents and apparatus.

2.3   Titrate according to the proposed experimental program. Pay attention to the preparation and calibration of the standard solution.

2.4   Design the form to record the original data, and then data processing. The total content of calcium and magnesium in the eggshell is expressed as the mass percentage of CaO.

3. Prompt

3.1   The main component of eggshell is $CaCO_3$, followed by $MgCO_3$, protein, pigment and a small amount of iron and aluminum.

3.2   First roughly determine the calcium and magnesium content in eggshell powder, and then estimate the weighing range of eggshell powder.

3.3   In general, calcium and magnesium in eggshell need be turned into ion form by heating and dissolving in the diluted acid. If there are some insoluble compounds, such as protein in solution, it does not affect the result of titration.

3.4   Due to the presence of protein, there is a small amount of foam on the surface of solution when preparing the sample solution. You can use a glass rob dipped a small amount of ethanol to touch and eliminate the foam.

3.5   Three kinds of titration analysis can be used respectively to determine the calcium and magnesium contents in the eggshell.

3.5.1　EDTA complex titration

In pH = 10 buffer solution, with chrome black T as an indicator and EDTA standard solution as a titrant, the content of calcium and magnesium can be determined by EDTA titration. Triethanolamine, a masking agent, is added before titration to eliminate the interference of Fe^{3+} and Al^{3+} on the measurement of Ca^{2+} and Mg^{2+}.

3.5.2　Acid-base titration

The carbonate in eggshell react with hydrochloric acid and excess hydrochloric acid can be back titrated using NaOH standard solution. According to the amount of hydrochloric acid reacted with $CaCO_3$, the content of calcium and magnesium in the eggshell are obtained.

3.5.3　Potassium permanganate titration

First, turn the calcium and magnesium in eggshell into ion form. Then these ions react with oxalic acid to formed oxalate precipitation. After filtration and washing, the precipitate is dissolved in acid solution. Then determine the $C_2O_4^{2-}$ content in the solution by potassium permanganate titration. According to the $C_2O_4^{2-}$ content, the content of calcium and magnesium in eggshell can be calculated.

4. Questions

4.1　How to determine the weighing range of eggshell powder?

4.2　Why the solutions of eggshell powder produce foam when diluting? How to eliminate the foom?

第四部分 大型分析仪器仿真操作

实验三十一 气相色谱-质谱联用仪的仿真操作

一、实验概况

气相色谱以氢气或其他可用气体为载气，对可挥发性有机化合物在气相色谱中进行高效分离。气相色谱柱的末端连接质谱仪，由于样品中各组分在气相色谱中已经得到高效的分离，各个谱带进入质谱被检测，得出每一扫描时间内的质谱图以及总离子流强度色谱图。对得到的谱图可以通过计算机自动谱库进行检索定性，还可以根据总离子流色谱图的峰高或峰面积定量。

二、实验装置

分析仪器仿真软件 ISTS 2.0（北京东方模拟软件科技有限公司）。

三、实验操作

1. 打开软件及实验前准备 启动 Ad500u.exe，选择"分析实验：气质联用"按钮，进入初始界面。点击仪器图片进入流程图界面。点击"实验前的准备"按钮，按照提示，进行步骤的排序，然后点击"确定"按钮，进入开机及调谐界面。顺次点击页码"1"～"5"，阅读注意事项。

2. 编辑实验方法 返回流程图界面，点击"切换至方法编辑"进入方法编辑界面。单击 Method 菜单中的"Load…"按钮，选择"30.M"文件并单击 OK。然后点击进入 Method/Edit Entire Method…窗口，选定三个选项，然后单击 OK。按照提示依次设置"进样源""压力单位""载气类型""进样口温度""分流比""载气平均速度""载气初始温度""柱温箱升温过程""扫描范围""threshold 值"和"样品率"参数，并选择"atune.u"作为调谐文件，选择"Percent Report"为报告方式，设定"Screen"为输出装置，单击 OK 按钮完成设置，并保存方法文件，返回到流程图界面。

3. 进样 点击"开始进样"进入自动进样界面，观看自动进样录像，然后点击进样器和主面板的"start"键。返回到进样界面。

4. 数据采集 点击"进入数据采集"按钮，演示数据采集过程，当出现"数据采集完毕"提示框，点击"确定"。

5. 数据分析　点击"开始数据分析"按钮进入数据分析界面。点击波峰（色谱峰），出现对应化合物的质谱棒图。右键双击质谱图，进行谱库检索，检索完成后，匹配结果会自动产生。

6. 实验结束　点击"实验结束"按钮，按照提示，依次关闭实验仪器的开关。

Experiment 31   Gas Chromatography Mass Spectrometry (GC–MS)

1. Experiment Overview

Use helium or other available gas as a carrier gas for efficient separation of volatile organic compounds by gas chromatography. The end of the GC column is connected to a mass spectrometer. Since each component in the sample has been efficiently separated in the gas chromatograph, each band enters the mass spectrum to be examined to obtain a mass spectrogram. Meanwhile, a total ion chromatogram is obtained. The quantitation can be based on the peak height or peak area of the total ion chromatogram.

2. Experimental Device

Analytical instrument simulation software ISTS 2.0 (Beijing East Simulation Software Technology Co., Ltd).

3. Experimental Operation

3.1   Start the software and prepare for the experiment

Start Ad500u.exe, select "Analyze Experiment: GC-MS" in the Training Project page, and click on the instrument image to enter the flow chart window. Then click the "Experiment Preparation" button. According to the tips, sort the experimental steps, and then click "OK" button to enter the boot window and tune window. Click the page number "1" to "5" to read the precautions.

3.2   Edit the experimental method

Return to the flowchart window and click "Switch to Method Edit" to enter the method editing window. Click the "Load..." button in the "Method" menu, select the "30.M" file and click OK. Then click into the "Method/Edit Entire Method..." window, select the three options, then click OK. Follow the prompts to set the parameters including "injection source" "pressure unit", "carrier gas type", "inlet temperature", "split ratio", "average carrier gas velocity", "carrier gas initial temperature", "column temperature", "heating process", "Scan range", "threshold value" and "sample rate", and select "atune.u" as the tuning file, select "Percent Report" as the reporting mode, and set "Screen" as the output device. Click the OK button to complete the setup and save the method file. Return to the flowchart window.

3.3 Injection

Click "Start Injection" to enter the auto-injection window and watch the auto-injection recording. Click the "start" button on the injector and main panel. Return to the injection window.

3.4 Data collection

Click the "Enter Data Acquisition" button to demonstrate the data collection process. When the "Data Acquisition Completed" prompt box appears, click OK.

3.5 Data analysis

Click the "Start Data Analysis" button to enter the data analysis window. Click on the peak and the mass spectrum bar graph of the corresponding compound appears. Click the right mouse button to perform a library search. After the search is completed, the matching result will be automatically generated.

3.6 End of the experiment

Click the "End of Experiment" button and follow the prompts to turn off the experimental instrument.

实验三十二　红外光谱仪仿真操作

一、实验概述

光源发出的连续波长的红外光经干涉仪、样品室到达检测器，检测到的红外干涉图包含了光源全部频率和强度的信息。计算机将干涉图函数进行付立叶变换就可以计算出光信号的强度按频率的分布，即单光光谱。测试样品的单光光谱与背景单光光谱的比值就是我们所需要的百分透过率红外光谱图。

二、实验装置

分析仪器仿真软件 ISTS 2.0（北京东方模拟软件科技有限公司）。

三、实验操作

1. 打开软件及参数设置　启动 Ad500u.exe，选择"分析实验：红外光谱分析"按钮，进入初始界面。点击仪器图片进入流程图界面。点击"扫描次数"和"分辨率"按钮设置相关参数（注意：输入完参数后，敲击主键盘上的回车键，数据才能有效）。返回流程图界面。

2. 样品制作　点击"软件操作"按钮进入制样界面。按照软件提示演示固体、液体和气体样品的制样过程。

3. 测试样品　返回流程图界面。点击"软件操作"进入测试界面。点击工具栏里的"Collect"按钮，在下拉菜单中选择"Experiment setup…"，开启样品收集。依次收集背景谱图和样品谱图。

4. 谱图分析　点击工具栏中的"Analysis"按钮，在下拉菜单中选择"Library Setup"，调出谱库搜索界面。点击"Search"按钮，开始谱库搜索。

5. 实验结束　点击"实验结束"按钮，按照提示，依次关闭实验仪器的开关。

Experiment 32　Infrared Spectroscopy (IR)

1. Experiment Overview

The continuous wave of infrared light from the light source passes through the interferometer and the sample chamber to the detector. The detected infrared interference pattern contains information of the full frequency and intensity of the light source. The computer transforms the interferogram function by Fourier and calculates the intensity of the optical signal by frequency distribution, that is, single light spectrum. The ratio of the single light spectrum of the test sample to the single light spectrum of the background is the percentage transmittance infrared spectrum.

2. Experimental Device

Analytical instrument simulation software ISTS 2.0 (Beijing East Simulation Software Technology Co., Ltd).

3. Experimental Operation

3.1　Start the software and parameter settings

Start Ad500u.exe and select the "Analyze Experiment: Infrared Spectrum Analysis" button to enter the initial window. Click on the instrument image to enter the flowchart interface. Click the "Scans" and "Resolution" buttons to set the relevant parameters (Note: After entering the parameters, hit the Enter key on the main keyboard to make the data valid). Return to the flowchart interface.

3.2　Sample production

Click the "Software Operation" button to enter the sample preparation window. Follow the software prompts to demonstrate the preparation of solid, liquid, and gas samples.

3.3　Sample testing

Return to the flowchart interface. Click "Software Operation" to enter the test window. Click on the "Collect" button in the toolbar and select "Experiment setup..." from the drop-down menu to open the sample collection. The background spectrum and sample spectrum are collected in sequence.

3.4　Spectral analysis

Click the "Analysis" button in the toolbar and select "Library Setup" from the drop-down menu to bring up the library search interface. Click the "Search" button to start the library search.

3.5 End of the experiment

Click the "End of Experiment" button and follow the prompts to turn off the experimental instrument.

实验三十三 原子吸收分光光度计的仿真操作

一、实验概述

原子吸收分光光度分析法又称原子吸收光谱分析法,是根据物质产生的原子蒸气对特定波长的光的吸收作用来进行定量分析的。

与原子发射光谱相反,元素的基态原子可以吸收与其发射波长相同的特征谱线。当光源发射的某一特征波长的光通过原子蒸气时,原子中的外层电子将选择性地吸收该元素所能发射的特征波长的谱线,这时,透过原子蒸气的入射光将减弱,其减弱的程度与蒸气中该元素的浓度成正比,吸光度符合吸收定律:

$$A = \lg (I_0/I) = K_c L$$

根据这一关系可以用工作曲线法或标准加入法来测定未知溶液中某元素的含量。

在火焰原子吸收光谱分析中,分析方法的灵敏度、准确度、干扰情况和分析过程是否简便快速等,除与所用仪器有关外,在很大程度上取决于实验条件。因此最佳实验条件的选择是个重要的问题。本实验在对钠元素测定时,分别对灯电流、狭缝宽度、燃烧器高度、燃气和助燃气流量比(助燃比)等因素进行选择。

二、实验装置

分析仪器仿真软件 ISTS 2.0(北京东方模拟软件科技有限公司)。

三、实验操作

1. 打开软件 启动 Ad500u.exe,选择"原子吸收"按钮,进入主界面。

2. 开机 点击原子吸收分光光度计,在出现的原子吸收分光放大图中点击右下角的总电源开关,打开电源。返回主界面。

3. 打开空气压缩机电源开关 点击空气压缩机,在出现的空气压缩机窗口点击电源开关,打开电源。返回主界面。

4. 选择阴极灯 点击原子吸收分光光度计,在出现的原子吸收分光光度计放大图中点击左上的阴极灯箱,出现阴极灯窗口。根据待测元素的不同选择相应的元素灯。然后点击阴极灯电源开关接通电源。返回原子吸收分光光度计放大图界面。

5. 粗调节阴极的灯电流 点击原子吸收分光光度计上的阴极灯电流指示位置,出现阴极灯电流调节窗口。在调节旋钮上点击鼠标左键增大电流,点击右键减小电流。根据实验要求,调节电流再 8～11 mA 之间。返回原子吸收分光光度计放大图界面。

6. 波长扫描 点击原子吸收分光光度计右下的波长扫描按钮。左边白色的按钮是在一定范围内自动从大到小扫描,灰色按钮是在一定范围内自动从小到大扫描。系统会自动扫描找到最合适的波长。

7. 调节多功能面板 点击原子吸收分光光度计右上的多功能面板,出现多功能面板的放大图。旋钮的旋转:鼠标左键点击逆时针旋转,鼠标右键点击顺时针旋转。调节"方式"到"调整"档。返回原子吸收分光光度计放大图界面。

8. 调节阴极灯位置 分别点击原子吸收分光光度计右下的能量表和阴极灯箱,打开能量表的放大图窗口和阴极灯调节窗口。分别在垂直和水平方向上调节阴极灯的位置,使得获得的能量最大,调节的时候一定要反复多试几次,如果在最大点位置附近移动一两下不好调准,可以先移动到最大点位置比较远的地方再向回调,如此反复几次,找准最大能量的位置。如果调整到最大能量后能量表指针偏出了红色区域,可以用增益旋钮调节使指针回到红色范围。调节好以后,关闭阴极灯窗口。不要关闭能量表窗口。

9. 微调波长 点击原子吸收分光光度计的波长微调旋钮,左键增加,右键减小,使获得最大的能量输出。如果调整到最大能量后能量表指针偏出了红色区域,可以用增益旋钮调节使指针回到红色范围。

10. 调节狭缝宽度 点击原子吸收分光光度计右上的多功能面板,用鼠标点击狭缝调节旋钮,左键点击顺时针旋转,右键点击逆时针旋转,调节需要的狭缝宽度。选择好狭缝宽度后,如果能量表的指针偏出红色区域,可以用增益旋钮调节使指针回到红色范围。调节好以后,关闭多功能面板和能量表窗口。返回到主界面。

11. 打开乙炔钢瓶 在主界面上点击乙炔钢瓶,会出现乙炔钢瓶的放大窗口。用鼠标左键点击乙炔总阀,总阀会自动打开。然后调节乙炔支阀,左键点击增加开度,右键点击减小开度,调节支压力表的压力到足够大,建议压力不小于 0.15 Mpa。调节完成后,关闭乙炔钢瓶窗口,回到主界面。

12. 接通气路、点火 在主界面上点击原子吸收分光光度计,出现原子吸收分光光度计放大图。点击原子吸收分光光度计的气路开关部分,出现气路开关放大的窗口,从左到右依次点击打开各个开关,然后关闭窗口,回到原子吸收分光光度计放大图界面。鼠标左键点住点火按钮几秒钟,火焰即被点燃。

13. 调零 打开原子吸收分光光度计多功能面板,点击"方式"旋钮使调整到"吸光度"位置后,关闭多功能面板。点击主界面右下的溶液烧杯选取溶液。选取"空白样液",并点击"确定"按钮,然后点击原子吸收分光光度计右下的调零按钮进行调零。

14. 调节燃烧器位置 任意选取一份在线性范围的标准对比样液。点击"确定"按钮自动喷入雾花器后,仪器会显示一定的吸光度值。然后点击原子分光光度计的燃烧器位置调节旋钮。两个旋钮中,上面的是调垂直位置(左键点击燃烧器向下移动,右键点击向上移动),下面的旋钮是调水平位置(键点击向右移动,右键点击向左移动)。调整的同时密切注意吸光度的变化,找到吸光度最大的位置。

15. 微调阴极灯电流 同时打开能量表窗口和阴极灯电流表窗口,调整阴极灯电流为 10 mA。如果调整电流后能量表指针偏出了红色区域,可以用增益旋钮调节使指针回到红色范围。调节好以后,关闭能量表窗口和阴极灯电流表窗口,返回原子吸收分光光度计放大图界面。

16. 调节空气和乙炔的流量 点击原子吸收分光光度计左下的空气和乙炔流量调节位置,出现空气和乙炔的流量调节窗口。先固定空气流量(具体值由实验确定),改变乙炔流量，使当前液指示吸光度最大。接着固定乙炔流量，改变空气流量，使当前液指示吸光度最大。关闭窗口。

17. 样品测试和数据记录　打开多功能面板，把"信号"旋钮转到"积分"位置。点击左边菜单的"溶液选取"或者"烧杯选择溶液"，依次测量各标准溶液和未知溶液，且在每次测试前都要用空白样液校零。每测量一种溶液后，点击"记录数据"按钮记录数据。

18. 数据处理　记录完最后一组数据后，点击"绘制曲线"按钮，出现绘制曲线界面。

19. 实验结束　点击"实验结束"按钮，按照提示，依次关闭实验仪器的开关。

Experiment 33　Atomic Absorption Spectrophotometer (AAS)

1. Experiment Overview

Atomic absorption spectrophotometry, also known as atomic absorption spectrometry, is a quantitative analysis of the absorption of light of a specific wavelength by the atomic vapor produced by a substance.

In contrast to atomic emission spectroscopy, the ground state atoms of the element can absorb the same characteristic emission line as their emission wavelength. When the light source emits a characteristic wavelength of light through the atomic vapor, the outer electron in the atom will selectively absorb the spectral wavelength of the characteristic wavelength that the element can emit. The incident light through the atomic vapor will be weakened and the extent of its attenuation is proportional to the concentration of the element in the vapor. Absorption in line with absorption law,

$$A = \lg (I_0/I) = K_c L$$

According to this relationship, the working curve method or standard addition method can be used to determine the content of some element in unknown solution.

In flame atomic absorption spectrometry, the sensitivity, accuracy, interference conditions and ease of analysis of analytical methods, etc., depend largely on the experimental conditions, except for the equipment involved. Therefore, the choice of the best experimental conditions is an important issue. In this experiment of the determination of sodium, the lamp current, slit width, burner height, gas and co-combustion gas flow ratio (combustion ratio) and other factors will be chosen.

2. Experimental Device

Analytical instrument simulation software ISTS 2.0 (Beijing East Simulation Software Technology Co., Ltd).

3. Experimental Operation

3.1　Start the software
Start Ad500u.exe and select the "Atomic Absorption" button to enter the main window.
3.2　Turn on the main power
Click the image of atomic absorption spectrophotometer and then click the power switch in

the pop-up AAS window. Close this window to return the main window.

3.3 Turn on the air compressor power

Click the air compressor, the air compressor window will appear. Click the power switch. Return to the main window.

3.4 Selection of the cathode lamp

Click the image of atomic absorption spectrophotometer. Then click the cathode light box on the top left in the pop-up AAS window, the cathode lamp window will appear. Select the appropriate light according to the different elements to be tested. Then click the power switch to turn on the lamp. Close this window to return to the AAS window.

3.5 Adjustment of the cathode lamp current

Click on the cathode lamp current indicating position, cathode lamp current adjustment window will appear. Left-clicking the mouse on the adjustment knob increases the current and right-clicking reduces the current. According to the experimental requirements, adjust the current between $8\sim11$ mA. Then close the current adjustment window and return to the AAS window.

3.6 Scan of the wavelength

Click the "scan the wavelength" button in the lower right corner. The system will find the most suitable wavelength.

3.7 Adjustment of multi-function panel

Click the multi-function panel in the upper right corner to display an enlarged view of the multi-function panel. Left click on the control knob for the counterclockwise rotation and right click on the control knob for the clockwise rotation. Adjust "Mode" to "Adjustment". Then close the multi-function panel to return to the AAS window.

3.8 Adjustment of the cathode lamp position

Click on the energy meter and cathode light box at the bottom right of AAS window to open the window of the energy meter and cathode lamp adjustment window. Adjust the position of the cathode lamp in vertical and horizontal directions, respectively, to obtain the maximum energy. If you adjust the maximum energy meter pointer out of the red area, you can use the gain knob to adjust the pointer back to the red range (Click the wavelength tuning knob, left to increase, right to reduce, so that the maximum energy output). After adjusting, close the cathode lamp window. Do not close the energy meter window.

3.9 Fine tune the wavelength

Click on the multi-function panel on the upper right of the AAS window to show the multi-function panel window. Click the wavelength adjustment knob to obtain the maximum energy output. The left button is increased and the right button is decreased. If the energy meter pointer is out of the red area after adjusting, you can use the gain knob to adjust the pointer back to the red range.

3.10 Adjustment of the slit width

Click on the slit adjustment knob, left-click clockwise rotation, and right-click counterclockwise rotation. If the pointer of the energy meter deviates from the red area, you can use the gain knob to adjust the pointer back to the red range. After adjustment, close the multi-function panel and the energy meter window, and then return to the main window.

3.11   Open the acetylene cylinder

Click "Acetylene cylinders" on the main window to show the enlarged acetylene cylinders window. Click on the acetylene main valve to open the main valve. Then adjust the pressure of the branch pressure gauge to large enough. The recommended pressure is not less than 0.15 Mpa. After complete the adjustment, close the acetylene cylinder window and return to the main window.

3.12   Processing and ignition

Click the image of atomic absorption spectrophotometer to show AAS window. Then click the gas switch on the middle lower part of AAS to show the enlarged window of the gas switch. Click left to right to open each switch, and then close this window to return the AAS window. Click the ignition button for a few seconds with the left mouse button and the flame is ignited.

3.13   Zero adjustment

Click the multifunction panel in the AAS window and click the "Mode" knob to adjust the "absorbance" position, and then close the multifunction panel. Click the "beaker" button in the main window to show a solution selection window. Select "blank sample solution" and then click the "OK" button. The selected solution will be sprayed into the nebulizer automatically. Click on the "zero button" to zero.

3.14   Adjust burner position

Select a sample of standard contrast in the linear range randomly. Click "OK" button. The instrument will display a certain absorbance value. Then click the burner position adjustment knob. While adjusting, pay close attention to the change of absorbance to find the position with the highest absorbance.

3.15   Fine-tune the cathode lamp current

Open windows of the energy meter and the cathode lamp current meter and adjust the value of current to 10 mA. If the energy meter pointer is out of the red area after adjusting the current, you can use the gain knob to adjust the pointer back to the red range. After adjustment, close the two windows.

3.16   Adjust the flow of air and acetylene

Click on the "air and acetylene flow adjustment" button on the AAS screen to show air and acetylene flow adjustment window. First, fix air flow (specific value determined experimentally), and change acetylene flow to make the absorbance maximum. Then fix acetylene flow, and change the air flow to make the absorbance maximum.

3.17   Sample testing and data logging

Open the multi-function panel and turn the "Signal" knob to the "Integral" position (As the absorbance value is constantly changing, turning the "Signal" knob to the "Signal Integral" can make the rate of change slower). Click on the left menu "solution selection" or "beaker" button to select the solution. Measure the standard solution and unknown solution sequentially. Before each test, use a blank sample solution to zero. After each test, click the "Record Data" button to record the data.

3.18 Data processing

After recording the last group of data, click on the "Draw Curves" button, the drawing curve window appears.

3.19 End of the experiment

Click the "End of Experiment" button and follow the prompts to turn off of the experimental instrument.

实验三十四　高效液相色谱的仿真操作

一、实验概述

以液体做流动相的色谱称为液相色谱。人们把已经比较成熟的气相色谱理论应用于液相色谱，使液相色谱得到了迅速的发展。随着其他科学技术的发展，出现了新型的高压输液泵、高效的固定相和柱填充技术、高灵敏度的检测器，加上计算机的应用，使得液相色谱实现了高效率和高速度。这种分离效率高、分析速度快的液相色谱称为高效液相色谱。

二、实验装置

分析仪器仿真软件 ISTS 2.0（北京东方模拟软件科技有限公司）。

三、实验操作

1. 打开软件　启动 Ad500u.exe，选择"分析实验：液相色谱"按钮，进入主界面。

2. 开机和了解操作条件　点击"启动液相色谱仪"按钮打开 HPLC 的主电源。点击"实验操作条件"按钮显示该模拟操作的标准操作条件。（注意：在模拟操作过程中，请根据本列表中的标准条件设置实验参数，否则色谱图将不会正确输出。）

3. 编辑色谱工作方法

（1）点击主界面上的计算机启动化学工作站。点击菜单"方法→编辑方法"，在弹出窗口中选择编辑内容。

（2）通过点击进样器、溶剂系统、色谱柱、检测器等图标，打开各部分的参数编辑窗口，按照实验要求的参数进行编辑，并采用"另存为"的方式保存方法。返回主页面。

4. 溶剂脱气　点击泵系统的 Purge 阀进行溶剂脱气，待试剂瓶的导管没有气泡流出，再次点击 Purge 阀结束脱气。

5. 样品测试

（1）点击主界面窗口左下角的"化学工作站"按钮进入化学工作站窗口。点击"打开系统"按钮，待状态指示栏变为绿色并显示"Ready"后，表明系统已经准备完毕，开始进行样品测试。

（2）点击"Start"或运行方法，然后点击试剂瓶开始自动进样。

（3）进样后，色谱显示区会出现色谱图，待色谱图出完后，样品分析完毕。

6. 报告实验结果　点击化学工作站界面上的"报告"按钮调出实验报告。根据得出的保留时间、峰高、半峰宽等实验数据，可以计算分离度等相关参数。也可点击右上角"打印报表"按钮打印实验报告。

7. 结束实验　点击"结束实验"按钮，然后关闭仪器。

Experiment 34　High Performance Liquid Chromatography (HPLC)

1. Experiment Overview

Chromatography using liquid as the mobile phase is called liquid chromatography. Applied the more mature theory of gas chromatography, the liquid chromatography has developed rapidly. With the development of other science and technology, such as new high-pressure infusion pumps, efficient stationary phase, technologies of column packing, high-sensitivity detectors and computer applications, liquid chromatography show high efficiency and high speed. This kind of liquid chromatography with high separation efficiency and fast analytics is known as high performance liquid chromatography (HPLC).

2. Experimental Device

Analytical instrument simulation software ISTS 2.0 (Beijing East Simulation Software Technology Co., Ltd).

3. Experimental Operation

3.1　Start software

Start Ad500u.exe, select the "Analyze Experiment: Liquid Chromatography" button to enter the main window.

3.2　Power on and read operating conditions

Click the "Start Liquid Chromatograph" button to turn on the main power of the HPLC. Click the "Experimental Operating Conditions" button to display the standard operating conditions for the simulation. (Note: During the simulation operation, set the experimental parameters according to the standard conditions in this list, otherwise the chromatogram will not be output correctly.)

3.3　Edit the experimental method

3.3.1　Click the computer icon to enter Chemstation. Click "Method" in the top menu bar and then "Edit method..." from the drop-down menu to show the following window gives you the option to edit the contents of the method.

3.3.2　Click icons including the injector, solvent system, columns, detectors and other parts in the center of the ChemStation to pop up the corresponding windows of setting parameters. The parameters can be adjusted according to the experimental requirements. After editing the method, save the method by using "Save As". Return to the main page.

3.4　Degassing of system

Click the "Purge" valve. When there are no air bubbles to flow out in the reagent bottle, click the Purge valve again to finish the degassing.

3.5　Sample testing

3.5.1　Click "Chemstation" button to enter Chemstation window. Click "Turn on the system" button and wait until the status bar becomes green and shows "Ready".

3.5.2　Click "Start" button. Then click on the reagent bottle to start the automatic injection.

3.5.3　After injection, the chromatogram will appear in the chromatographic display area. After the chromatogram is finished, the sample is analyzed.

3.6　Output the experiment report

Click the "Report" button on the ChemStation screen to bring up the lab report. Based on the experimental data such as retention time, peak height, and half-width, the correlation parameters such as resolution can be calculated. You can also print an experiment report by clicking the "Print Report" button in the upper right corner.

3.7　End of the experiment

Click the "End of Experiment" button and follow the prompts to turn off of the experimental instrument.

第五部分　附　录

附录 1　常用指示剂

1. 酸碱指示剂（18~25 ℃）

指示剂	变色 pH 范围	颜色		配制方法	用量滴/10 ml
		酸色	碱色		
百里酚蓝	1.2~2.8	红	黄	0.1 g 指示剂溶于 100 ml 20%乙醇中	1~2
甲基黄	2.9~4.0	红	黄	0.1 g 指示剂溶于 100 ml 90%乙醇中	1
甲基橙	3.2~4.4	红	橙黄	0.1%水溶液	1
溴酚蓝	3.0~4.6	黄	紫	0.1 g 指示剂溶于 100 ml 20%乙醇中	1
溴甲酚绿	3.8~5.4	黄	蓝	0.1 g 指示剂溶于 100 ml 20%乙醇中	1
甲基红	4.2~6.3	红	黄	0.1 g 指示剂溶于 100 ml 60%乙醇中	1
溴百里酚蓝	6.2~7.6	黄	蓝	0.05 g 指示剂溶于 100 ml 20%乙醇中	1
中性红	6.8~8.0	红	亮黄	0.1 g 指示剂溶于 100 ml 60%乙醇中	1
酚红	6.7~8.4	黄	红	0.1 g 指示剂溶于 100 ml 60%乙醇中	1
酚酞	8.0~10.0	无	红	0.1 g 指示剂溶于 100 ml 60%乙醇中	1~3
百里酚酞	9.4~10.6	无	蓝	0.1 g 指示剂溶于 100 ml 90%乙醇中	1~2

2. 混合酸碱指示剂

指示剂的组成	变色点 pH	颜色		备注
		酸色	碱色	
一份 0.1%甲基黄乙醇溶液 一份 0.1%次甲基蓝乙醇溶液	3.25	蓝紫	绿	pH 3.2 蓝紫色 pH 3.4 绿色
一份 0.1%甲基橙溶液 一份 0.25%靛蓝（二甲黄）水溶液	4.1	紫	黄绿	pH 4.1 灰色
三份 0.1%溴甲酚绿乙醇溶液 一份 0.2%甲基红乙醇溶液	5.1	酒红	绿	颜色变化显著
一份 0.1%溴甲酚绿钠盐水溶液 一份 0.1%氯酚红钠盐水溶液	6.1	黄绿	蓝紫	pH 5.4 蓝绿色 pH 5.8 蓝色 pH 6.2 蓝紫

指示剂的组成	变色点 pH	颜色		备注
		酸色	碱色	
一份 0.1%中性红乙醇溶液 一份 0.1%次甲基蓝乙醇溶液	7.0	蓝紫	绿	pH 7.0 蓝紫
一份 0.1%甲酚红钠盐水溶液 三份 0.1%百里酚蓝钠盐水溶液	8.3	黄	紫	pH 8.2 玫瑰色 pH 8.4 紫色
一份 0.1%百里酚蓝 50%乙醇溶液 三份 0.1%酚酞 50%乙醇溶液	9.0	黄	紫	pH 9.0 绿色
二份 0.1%百里酚酞乙醇溶液 一份 0.1%茜素黄乙醇溶液	10.2	黄	紫	

3. 非水滴定指示剂

指示剂	颜色		配制方法
	酸色	碱色	
结晶紫	蓝、绿、黄	紫	0.5%冰 HAc 溶液
α-萘酚苯甲醇	绿	黄	0.5%冰 HAc 溶液
喹哪啶红	无	红	0.1%无水甲醇溶液
偶氮紫	蓝	红	0.1%二甲基甲酰胺溶液
百里酚蓝	蓝	黄	0.3%无水甲醇溶液
溴酚蓝	红	蓝	1%无水乙醇溶液

4. 金属离子指示剂

指示剂	pH 范围	颜色		配制方法
		In	MIn	
铬黑 T（EBT）	7～10	蓝	红	0.5%水溶液
二甲酚橙（XO）	<6	亮黄	蓝紫	0.2%水溶液
吡啶偶氮萘酚（PAN）	2～12	黄	红	0.1%乙醇溶液
钙指示剂（NN）	10～13	纯蓝	酒红	0.5%乙醇溶液

5. 氧化还原指示剂

指示剂名称	$\psi^{\theta'}$ [H$^+$]=1 mol/L	颜色变化		溶液配制方法
		氧化色	还原色	
中性红	0.24	红色	无色	0.05%的 60%乙醇溶液
次甲基蓝	0.36	蓝色	无色	0.05%的水溶液

指示剂名称	$\psi^{\theta'}$ [H$^+$]=1 mol/L	颜色变化		溶液配制方法
		氧化色	还原色	
变胺蓝	0.59（pH=2）	无色	蓝色	0.05%的水溶液
二苯胺	0.76	紫色	无色	1%的浓硫酸溶液
二苯胺磺酸钠	0.85	紫红色	无色	0.5%的水溶液
N-邻苯氨基苯甲酸	1.08	紫红色	无色	0.1 g 指示剂加 20 ml 5%的 Na$_2$CO$_3$ 溶液，用水稀释至 100 ml
邻二氮菲-Fe（Ⅱ）	1.06	浅蓝	红	1.485 g 邻二氮菲加 0.965 g FeSO$_4$，溶于 100 ml 水中（0.025 mol/L 水溶液）
5-硝基邻二氮菲-Fe（Ⅱ）	1.25	浅蓝	紫红	1.608 g 5-硝基邻二氮菲加 0.695 g FeSO$_4$，溶于 100 ml 水中（0.025 mol/L 水溶液）

6. 常用的吸附指示剂

指示剂	滴定剂	适用的 pH 范围	待测离子
荧光黄	Ag$^+$	7～10（常用 7～8）	Cl$^-$
二氯荧光黄	Ag$^+$	4～10（常用 5～8）	Cl$^-$
曙红	Ag$^+$	2～10（常用 3～9）	Br$^-$、I$^-$、SCN$^-$
甲基紫	Ba^{2+}、Cl$^-$	1.5～3.5	SO$_4^{2-}$、Ag$^+$
橙黄素Ⅳ 氨基苯磺酸 溴酚蓝	Ag$^+$	微酸性	Cl$^-$、I$^-$混合液及生物碱盐类
二甲基二碘荧光黄	Ag$^+$	中性	I$^-$

附录 2 常用缓冲溶液的配制

缓冲溶液组成	pK_a	缓冲液 pH	配制方法
甘氨酸 – HCl	2.35	2.3	取甘氨酸 15 g 溶于 50 ml 水中，加浓 HCl 8 ml，用水稀释至 100 ml
一氯乙酸 – NaOH	2.85	2.8	取 20 g 一氯乙酸溶于 20 ml 水中，加 NaOH 4 g 溶解后，用水稀释至 100 ml
甲酸 – NaOH	3.77	3.7	取 9.5 g 甲酸和 NaOH 4 g 溶于 50 ml 水中，溶解后用水稀释至 100 ml
HAc – NaAc	4.76	4.6	取 8.3 g 无水 NaAc 溶于 50 ml 水中，加冰 HAc 6 ml，用水稀释至 100 ml
$NaH_2PO_4 – Na_2HPO_4$	7.21（pK_{a_1}）	6.8	取 0.2 mol/L 磷酸二氢钾溶液 250 ml，加 0.2 mol/L 氢氧化钠溶液 118 ml，用水稀释至 1000 ml，摇匀，即得
$NaH_2PO_4 – Na_2HPO_4$	7.21（pK_{a_1}）	7.2	取 0.2 mol/L 磷酸二氢钾溶液 50 ml 与 0.2 mol/L 氢氧化钠溶液 35 ml，加新沸过的冷水稀释至 200 ml，摇匀，即得
Tris – HCl	8.21	8.2	取 25 g Tris 试剂溶于水中，加 HCl 8 ml，稀释至 1 L
$NH_3 – NH_4Cl$	9.26	8.0	取 NH_4Cl 1.07 g 加水使溶解成 100 ml，再加稀氨溶液（1→30）调节 pH 至 8.0，加水稀释至 1 L
$NH_3 – NH_4Cl$	9.26	10	取氯化铵 5.4 g，加水 20 ml 溶解后，加浓氨溶液 35 ml，再加水稀释至 100 ml，即得

附录 3 0～95 ℃时标准缓冲溶液的 pH

温度 ℃	(1) 0.05 mol/L 邻苯二甲酸氢钾	(2) 0.025 mol/L KH$_2$PO$_4$ + 0.025 mol/L K$_2$HPO$_4$	(3) 0.08695 mol/L KH$_2$PO$_4$ + 0.03043 mol/L K$_2$HPO$_4$	(4) 0.01 mol/L 硼砂	(5) 25 ℃饱和氢氧化钙
0	4.003	6.984	7.534	9.464	13.423
5	3.999	6.951	7.500	9.395	13.207
10	3.998	6.923	7.472	9.332	13.003
15	3.999	6.900	7.448	9.276	12.810
20	4.002	6.881	7.429	9.225	12.627
25	4.008	6.865	7.413	9.180	12.454
30	4.015	6.853	7.400	9.139	12.289
35	4.024	6.844	7.389	9.102	12.133
38	4.030	6.840	7.384	9.081	12.043
40	4.035	6.838	7.380	9.068	11.984
45	4.047	6.834	7.373	9.038	11.841
50	4.060	6.833	7.367	9.011	11.705
55	4.075	6.834	……	8.985	11.574
60	4.091	6.836	……	8.962	11.449
70	4.126	6.845	……	8.921	……
80	4.164	6.859	……	8.885	……
90	4.205	6.877	……	8.850	……
95	4.227	6.886	……	8.833	……

附录4 常用酸碱的密度、含量和浓度

试剂名称	密度（g/ml）	含量	浓度
盐酸	1.18～1.19	36～38	11.6～12.4
硝酸	1.39～1.40	65.0～68.0	14.4～15.2
硫酸	1.83～1.84	95～98	17.8～18.4
磷酸	1.69	85	14.6
高氯酸	1.68	70.0～72.0	11.7～12.0
冰醋酸	1.05	99.8（优级纯）	17.4
		99.0（分析纯、化学纯）	
氢氟酸	1.13	40	22.5
氢溴酸	1.49	47.0	8.6
氨水	0.88～0.90	25.0～28.0	13.3～14.8

参考文献

[1] 严拯宇，杜迎翔. 分析化学实验与指导 [M]. 3 版. 北京：中国医药科技出版社，2015.

[2] 王少云，姜维林. 分析化学与药物分析实验 [M]. 济南：山东大学出版社，2004.

[3] 柴逸峰，邸欣. 分析化学 [M]. 8 版. 北京：人民卫生出版社，2016.

[4] 朱明芳. 分析化学实验 [M]. 北京：科学出版社，2016.

[5] 邓湘舟. 现代分析化学实验 [M]. 北京：化学工业出版社，2013.

[6] 孙毓庆. 分析化学实验 [M]. 北京：科学出版社，2004.

[7] 李发美. 分析化学 [M]. 7 版. 北京：人民卫生出版社，2011.

参考文献

[1] 李洪心. 口腔解剖生理学实验指导[M]. 北京：人民卫生出版社，2015.

[2] 皮昕. 口腔解剖生理学[M]. 北京：人民卫生出版社，2004.

[3] 王美青. 口腔解剖生理学[M]. 8版. 北京：人民卫生出版社，2015.

[4] 王松灵. 牙体解剖学[M]. 北京：科学出版社，2016.

[5] 郑麟蕃. 现代口腔医学[M]. 北京：科学出版社，2000.

[6] 邱蔚六. 口腔医学[M]. 北京：世界图书出版公司，2004.

[7] 赵士杰. 口腔解剖学[M]. 北京：北京大学医学出版社，2011.